D1072438

Issues in Brain/Behavior Control

Issues in Brain/Behavior Control

Edited by
W. Lynn Smith, Ph.D.
Director, Cortical Function Laboratory
Porter Memorial Hospital
Denver, Colorado
and
Department of Biological Sciences
University of Denver

and

Arthur Kling, M.D.
Department of Psychiatry
Rutgers Medical School
College of Medicine and Dentistry of New Jersey
Piscataway, New Jersey

S P Books Division of
SPECTRUM PUBLICATIONS, INC.
New York

Distributed by Halsted Press
A Division of John Wiley & Sons

New York Toronto London Sydney

To Sylva

and Rosalyn

SPECTRUM PUBLICATIONS, INC.
86-19 Sancho Street, Holliswood, N.Y. 11423

Distributed solely by the Halsted Press division of John Wiley & Sons, Inc., New York

Library of Congress Cataloging in Publication Data

Main entry under title:

Issues in brain/behavior control.

Papers presented at a symposium held in Coronado, Calif.
Includes index.
1. Aggressiveness (Psychology)–Congresses.
2. Violence–Congresses. 3. Psychosurgery–Congresses. 4. Brain–Congresses. I. Smith, Wallace Lynn, 1922- II. Kling, Arthur, 1929-
RC555.I78 616.8'584 76-4949
ISBN 0-470-15038-6

Contributors

JOSEPH E. BOGEN, M.D.
Senior Neurosurgeon
Ross-Loos Medical Group
Los Angeles, California

CARLOS CLIMENT
Universidad del Valle
Cali, Colombia

FRANK R. ERVIN, M.D.
Department of Psychiatry
School of Medicine
University of California
Los Angeles, California

ROBERT GRIMM, M.D.
Neurological Sciences Institute
Good Samaritan Medical Center
Portland, Oregon

ROGER F. JOHNSON, M.D., L.L.B.
Johnson and Mahoney, P.C.
Denver, Colorado

ARTHUR KLING, M.D.
Department of Psychiatry
Rutgers Medical School
Piscataway, New Jersey

ROBERT PLUTCHIK, PH. D.
Department of Psychiatry
Albert Einstein College of Medicine
Yeshiva University
Bronx, New York

SALEEM A. SHAH, PH. D.
Chief, Center for Studies of Crime and Delinquency
National Institute of Mental Health
Rockville, Maryland

W. LYNN SMITH, PH. D.
Director
Cortical Function Laboratory
Porter Memorial Hospital
Denver, Colorado

ELLIOT S. VALENSTEIN, PH. D.
Department of Psychology and Neuroscience Laboratory
University of Michigan
Ann Arbor, Michigan

Contents

Introduction

I wish to commend the contributors to this volume for their courage in participating in this conference, especially in the light of the highly controversial nature of the subject. Unfortunately, the very nature of this topic, brain/behavior control of violence, often makes it difficult for many to separate medical and scientific issues from political, social, and personal biases.

You will note in the following papers that individual attitudes are specifically expressed by the scheduled participants. Not noted was the demonstration by an unscheduled group of college students who displayed their objections over the meeting topic itself. Fortunately, as to the meeting, all went well and ended well. The symposium, I might add as its permanent chairman, was the fifth of an annual series on cerebral function and was held in Coronado, California, last year. This yearly event is a multidisciplinary gathering of neuroscientists who share common interests in brain/behavior correlates. We express our sincere gratitude to Hoffmann-La Roche, Inc. and Ives Laboratories, Inc., whose generous support made this meeting possible.

As a clinical neuropsychologist, I will try to place the problem of the neural regulation of aggressive behavior in perspective. Since the advent of modern neurophysiology, many of the most respected workers have been concerned with elucidating the anatomical, physiological, and biochemical substrates of aggressive behavior. One only has to recall the contributions of Reanson, Magoun, Bard, Mountcastle, Hess, Klüver, Rioch, Fulton and McLean, to recognize that there has been continuous research interest in this subject. Thus, we already know a good deal about the neural pathways and anatomical areas underlying the elicitation of aggressive behavior in sub-human species. To be sure, we may have only scratched the surface, and many of the older concepts and results will be re-evaluated in the light of more sophisticated techniques and understanding of behavioral mechanisms.

Before and during the early experiments on temporal lobe, the frontal lobotomy era began and ended, stimulated by the pioneering experiments of Fulton and Jacobson. It is probably true that the reason for the abrupt decline in frontal lobotomy was not entirely the disenchantment with the results but the advent of the major tranquilizing drugs as well. Had the introduction of these powerful psychotropic agents been delayed a decade or so, we would quite likely have seen continued use and refinement of those surgical procedures.

My co-editor of this volume, Professor Kling, as you may know, has been carrying out basic research on the function of the amygdaloid nucleus for over twenty years. It was Dr. Leon Schreiner and Dr. Kling who first demonstrated that the "Klüver-Bucy" syndrome, called temporal lobectomy, could be produced by lesions of only the amygdaloid nucleus. A score of years ago no thought was given to applying the results of these experiments to human neurological or psychiatric problems. Since these early studies, however, a great deal of research into the functions of limbic system structures was conducted and continues, here and abroad.

Interestingly, the discussion in this volume has largely ignored the continuing use of selective lesions of the frontal lobe in man and has focused on the amygdalotomy procedure and more particularly on the 13 cases reported by Drs. Mark and Ervin, as if the amygdala, by virtue of its location deep in the medial surface of the hemisphere, is somehow closer to the abstract concept "soul". However, what has emerged from the study of the human split-brain series is that the "soul" is not likely to be found in any one location. Early studies in commissurotomized patients led one neurosurgeon to believe that the splenium might well be the seat of the soul, since patients in which it was spared did much better post-operatively. Yet with further cases, an almost hierarchical involvement has been noted which now includes the splenium as well as the reticular activating system and the limbic system, although the RAS undoubtedly remains at the top of the heap. Most of us are relieved that we need no longer entertain the pineal body. So much for soul searching.

One of the major themes of this conference is the question of the control of aggressive or violent behavior. Few would disagree today that "aggressive behavior", in the broadest sense, is built into the nervous system and is required for the survival of the species. A lack of "aggression", or striving, is coincident with individual and social deterioration and eventual dissolution of the group or society.

Given an opportunity in appropriate circumstances, Dr. Kling reminds us, all primates including man will utilize a variety of distance communication to avoid direct physical combat. Disturbances in brain function which may result in inappropriate and increased aggressive or violent behavior may be the result of increased discharges from brain areas facilitating aggressive behavior (amygdala, hypothalamus, brain stem). Critical damage to inhibitory structures or disturbances to brain areas resulting in disordered communication lead to physical means of communication and frequent combat.

Any of these groups of disorders may be facilitated or attenuated by social, environmental factors as well as by personality disorders interacting with the above. Thus there is a dire need for research into the influence of these factors on established brain dysfunction.

Perhaps the most beneficial result of this conference will be the generation of research into these vitally important problems.

In introducing this conference, Dr. Bogen has raised a number of knotty questions of definitions, or responsibility for treatment, as well as quality and appropriatness of treatment programs for individuals suffering from behavior disorders with varying etiologies. Each of these questions would require far more extensive discussion than was available within the scope of this conference. While some of these issues were ably discussed by the contributors, it is obvious that we are a long way from closure.

In this symposium, Dr. Valenstein has pointed to problems inherent in utilizing electrical stimulation. While lesion studies also have inherent problems, they should not hinder further investigation, but be a stimulus for better solutions. Continued and increased research by neuroscientists and clinicians is essential and should not be deterred by those who see possible misapplication of this information. Dr. Grimm has discussed this potential as well as the misuse of drugs and other forms of psychiatric intervention. As knowledge of brain mechanisms expands we will be able rationally to evaluate proposed experimental procedures applied to man instead of having only opinions and beliefs based on inadequate data. We need vastly improved methods of evaluating human behavioral function related to brain mechanisms, especially those concerned with behaviors occuring in a social context. Dr. Plutchik has presented the results of an attempt to develop a research methodology to identify factors related to violent behavior as well as a set of psychometric tools for further research.

Dr. Ervin has described a sub-population of individuals who are repeatedly involved in acts of personal violence and who have symptoms suggestive of an epileptic disorder. Dr. Plutchik's findings tend partially to support this contention in that he finds a high probability of people with focal epilepsy suffering from dyscontrol syndromes; however, their behavioral disorder does not involve violence. Rather, the high incidence of violence occurs in those who are already identified from prison populations and who have a history of family violence and who are schizoid or frankly psychotic. Dr. Grimm regards rage as being largely independent of the temporal lobe or limbic system paroxysmal disorders.

In the planning stages of this volume I had several inquiries regarding the person with XYY chromosomal abnormality, especially in reference to violence. One common misconception was in the Speck case. Although this genetic anomaly is not directly related to the topic of brain/behavior control, the interest is such as to necessitate a definitive discussion by a leading authority in this area. Dr. Shah has critically examined the XYY chromosomal abnormality as a predisposing genetic defect in aggressive behavior. His results point out the lack of evidence for relating this defect to violent behavior.

The papers in this book are multidisciplinary, overlapping and somewhat difficult to integrate, but several major questions emerge concerning technology, ethics and social responsibility.

Who is responsible for treatment of violent-aggressive persons? Are neurosurgical procedures, although still innovative, an appropriate treatment, even in specifically selected patients? What are the possible side effects of iatrogenic brain damage? On which patients should such procedures be conducted and under what conditions? What legal safeguards are necessary or desirable? What are the implications for future research and treatment of seriously ill people in light of the recent court rulings? Who will decide these issues in our society? Those who will ultimately decide these issues will be the ultimate controllers. Then who will control the controllers?

Answers to these questions will affect not only those directly associated with neurosurgical procedures and behavior, but also electrode implantation, psychopharmacotherapy and all other forms of psychologically induced methods of behavior control.

As Dr. Grimm put it so well, "As we approach our 200th birthday as a nation, brain control should be an 'open agenda', a public issue, informed, argumentative, with all being heard". Amen.

W. Lynn Smith, Ph.D.

Some Questions, Assumptions and Problems Involved in Associating Dyssocial Behavior with Disorders of Cerebral Function.

JOSEPH E. BOGEN
Senior Neurosurgeon
Ross-Loos Medical Group
Los Angeles, California

Like the rest of you here, I have been embroiled in a good many discussions over the past few years on such subjects as giving amphetamines to the child who misbehaves in the school room, using large doses of phenothiazines for the adult who is flagrantly schizophrenic, or advising psychosurgery for those of any age who are recurrently assaultive. Several conclusions seem to be inescapable: First, that most of us harbor very strong convictions, or at least intense feelings, on such subjects; second, that the differences of opinion among us stem both from differences in our experiences and from differences in how we understand the words with which we argue; and third, that it is usually quite difficult to reach agreement even on a precise specification of what it is we are arguing about. It is a fact of my own recent experience, for example, that many of those who are opposed to psychosurgery are also opposed to any attempt to define it (1).

If we can make only a little progress in the direction of definition and particularization, this symposium will probably have been justified.

Therefore, I should like to suggest at the start what some of the more sticky issues, questions or problems might be. Hopefully, as the symposium unfolds further, it will become clearer to us which of these problems are amenable to constructive discussion and which are not.

What do we understand by "cerebral function"? Does all speech depend upon cerebral function? I suppose so; but is this true of *any* behavior? Surely not, for we know that many a relatively simple form of behavior—for example, immediate withdrawal from a noxious stimulus—occurs about as often, and in the same way, with or without the cerebrum. On the other hand, when behavior is more complex, when it involves sizable delays in responding or involves responses whose form seems related to previous experience, then we usually conclude that the cerebrum *is* involved. Can we consider it a general rule that the more complex or less stimulus-bound an activity is, the more important is the cerebral contribution? When we come to what are often considered the highest functions—as, for example, imagination, foresight, altruistic love, creativity and the like—have we concurrently come to those functions which are the most dependent on the cerebrum? Most of us here would probably say yes. But we must admit that this is an unproved faith. And we must recognize that higher mental activity which is in some way independent of cerebral function is an aspect of the faith of some very eminent neuroscientists (2,3). Does this difference between two unproved faiths underlie some of the arguments which purport to concern more mundane matters?

Let us pass on to a question that is hardly any easier: What is "dyssocial behavior"? Is it any behavior which you or I individually find disagreeable or threatening? Or shall we take a vote, and then define as "dyssocial" any behavior which is disapproved by a slim majority temporarily existing at the time of balloting? Or should we depend on the individual himself? Perhaps we do not have to vote or otherwise define what we mean, so long as the particular individual himself considers his own behavior to be undesirable. But this is no solution—we must still form an opinion of our own before we can consider the inevitable issues of whether the individual in question is being self-punitive or self-deluding.

How about the individual who is self-destructive? Where self-destructiveness is as flagrant as in the Lesch-Nyhan syndrome,* a diagnosis of cerebral dysfunction is hardly arguable—but is it correct

*A combination including gout, mental retardation and self-mutilation (including the eating of one's own lips) which results from an hereditary enzyme defect (hypoxanthine-guanine phosphoribosyltransferase). See reference 3a.

to call such behavior "dyssocial"? Is it either dyssocial or mentally abnormal to self-mutilate in order to obtain some secondary goal, such as avoiding a military draft? If not, how about the self-mutilation of the Munchausen syndrome,* where the goals are poorly if at all defined?

What we mean by "dyssocial" is in some respects related to what we mean by "illegal." What do these two have in common, and—more interesting—how are they different? Hopefully Dr. Roger Johnson will help us with this among other questions.

Well, let us suppose that we have momentarily satisfied ourselves as to what constitutes "dyssocial behavior" and that we are also prepared to grant the brain a basic role in behavioral control. We would still be far from concluding that a particular dyssocial act is *best* understood in neurologic terms. Even when the brain is obviously diseased, it is often far from obvious that this disease is an important cause of the dyssocial behavior.

When there is a big earthquake and lots of people start running around like headless chickens, we suppose that their nervous systems are less stable or less adaptive in some way than the brains of people who are still acting purposefully in spite of the disaster. But we do not emphasize this brain difference so much as we emphasize the external cause. In most clinical practice, such persons are said to be suffering from a "transient situational reaction." Although mild tranquilizers might be in order, we mainly believe that the best solutions are to be found in some social remedy, perhaps even in something as simple as giving them hot food or a place to sleep or someone to talk to who is less frightened then they are.

What if the social dislocation is more chronic, such as being kept in a threatening environment interminably? Who was crazy in *Catch-22*—Yossarian or the system in which he was stuck? Perhaps Dr. Arthur Kling will provide us with some pointers on how to ascribe a proper proportion of causation to whatever is inside an individual rather than to what is outside of him.

Let us suppose that we have all agreed (some supposition!) that there are instances when an individual has indeed acted dyssocially, and that it is mostly because his particular brain is not functioning optimally. How vigorously he should be treated would then depend upon the severity of his disorder. How many acts of self-destruction

*A comprehensive account of this complicated syndrome (4) is not possible in a single sentence. Briefly, the patient presents repeatedly at different hospitals with ingeniously contrived, self-inflicted and difficult-to-diagnose disabilities; he does this presumably to obtain the food, lodging, narcotics and attention often made available for extended periods to "interesting cases."

must he commit to finally reach the magic number? Perhaps we can analogize with epilepsy: one seizure *does not* make a person epileptic. There must be, by definition, *recurrent* seizures. How many does this mean? At least four? Six? A dozen? It is the practice of some to say that surgery for epilepsy should be considered when, under the best medical management, the patient continues to have at least one daytime seizure per month for at least six months. Is this number appropriate for assaultive behavior? That is, shall we only make the diagnosis of "intractable episodic assaultive behavior" when an individual commits at least one seemingly unprovoked assault per month for at least six months? Should we really wait that long while the victims accumulate? If not, what number shall we use? Or is it sensible at all to look for a particular number as a measure of the propensity for dyssocial behavior? Perhaps Dr. Frank Ervin can suggest some criteria for this sort of problem.

Let us suppose that we have all agreed that something should be done without waiting much longer. Which procedure we advocate will probably depend upon which procedure we happen to have learned. Surgeons are gung ho for surgery, the psychotherapists love to listen (and talk), the behavior therapists have their thing, and so on. Therapeutic conferences are often reminiscent of the old story that if you give a little boy a hammer, it is absolutely amazing how almost everything in sight seems to need a healthy hammering! Would it really be any better to give him a screw driver? What if we gave our hypothetical child an extensive and diversified toolkit—would he then do less damage? Or maybe even more?

Perhaps, if we are sufficiently eclectic and simultaneously well-balanced (and aren't we all, those of us here?), our choice of treatment will not depend upon accidents of education or upbringing, or upon local logistic convenience. Perhaps what we should do is to choose the procedure which seems least irreversible. That seems sensible. In other words, having agreed that there is a problem needing action, we should do the simplest things first. Then if necessary we can progress in some systematic fashion to the more costly, then to the more unpleasant, then to the more risky, and then to the more definitely damaging. And all the while we will be hoping that some impressive success will soon appear and thus obviate the need for going further down the line.

In order to try various remedies in their proper order, we must first order them by some measure of their hazards. For example, when we consider how much cerebral damage a procedure can cause, surely our evaluation of the results should include thorough, skilled psychological testing (5, 6).* But as a prominent psychologist (not of the present company) recently said to me with respect to psychological testing, "No matter who does what tests, somebody will find them wanting." What can we do about that? Has Dr. Robert Plutchik some answers for us here?

And have any of you had the experience which I have had, that those who are the most insistent that therapy should await truly scientific evaluation of results are often persons with little or no therapeutic responsibility?

Let us move along, having assumed for the moment that we can assign costs and risks with a sufficient confidence. Nowadays, most persons with a severe pain problem would choose analgesics before acupuncture, alcohol injections before cordotomy, and cingulotomy before frontal lobotomy. But such an ascending series should hardly include *everything* for *every* problem. Nobody would interpose cordotomy before doing a cerebral operation if the problem were assaultive or other compulsive behavior. Even when the risks are restricted to loss of time, who wants to waste time trying acupuncture for a suicidal depression? Perhaps I exaggerate. But the general point is surely correct: if something does not work, an estimate of its risks and costs is irrelevant. If my advance information is correct, Dr. Elliot Valenstein will be addressing himself to this question of the efficacy, if any, of various procedures.

What do we mean when we say that something "works"? Do we mean that it usually makes people better? Well, then, what is "better"? More docile? Less complaining? When someone with widespread spinal metastases screams in pain every time he tries to turn in bed, docility seems heaven-sent.

But more generally we take a different view—the view that an individual is better, not when his behavioral repertoire has been reduced, but rather when it has been expanded. A conditioning procedure which eventuates in some stereotyped response is *not* what we are looking for. Consider *Clockwork Orange*, in which the protagonist is conditioned to retch whenever he sees the bare bod. This is considered preferable to what he used to do, which was to consider rape whenever he was in that situation. That he is accidentally conditioned at the same time to retch when he hears

*In this connection we may note that failure to report psychometric results has brought scathing criticism from his colleagues (7) on at least one neurosurgeon. And failure to consider relevant neurologic aspects has brought sharp criticism from a fellow psychoanalyst (8) on another author. Such examples do indeed suggest a need for a broader eclecticism.

Beethoven completely misses the point and is in fact a serious novelistic flaw, because it confuses the issue. What if this side effect had not occurred? Would the treatment then have been a success? I think not. Retching is less dyssocial than rape, but what a puny solution in which the patient's behavioral repertoire is no richer after treatment than it was before!

To be a better person one should be *more*, not less, differentiated (9). An automatic retching response to bare breasts is about as minimal a cerebral function as one can conceive. What one does who is really using his cerebrum in the presence of bifurcated beauty usually depends on *other* things—such as "Whose are they?" or "why are they bare?" (Or as one member of a group of nurses said when I used this example in a talk, "Yes—and how much time is there?").

Surely an essential measure of successful treatment is that it should usefully increase the patient's repertoire—that is, his capacity for choice.

When an individual is afflicted with some form of stereotyped behavior, its elimination may then provide him with an opportunity in which to consider other alternatives. But this will only be true if he has, somewhere along the line, accumulated a variety of different activities among which to choose.

No doubt the elimination of some repetitive, compulsive act will help to free the individual for the subsequent acquisition of alternative behaviors. I recall that when I decided some years ago never to strike my children for a trial period of one year, I subsequently felt almost powerless, especially in the beginning. Then, as time passed, it turned out that there are dozens of ways to cope, ways which came to me gradually over the months. By the end of the year I had such a large "armamentarium," as medical men are wont to call it, that I never again felt the need to resume corporal punishment. And now, in fact, I consider it a symptom of pedagogical impoverishment, or maybe even downright simple-mindedness.

But I want to emphasize that my new behavior pattern required not only forgoing an habitual solution, it also required the acquisition of other solutions. Trial and error alone will not suffice. The fact is, I had a lot of help in the form of advice from persons who already knew other ways to cope with children.

So shall we conclude that no doctor should ever undertake to eliminate a compulsion or any form of uncontrollable impulse unless he simultaneously commits himself to the subsequent rehabilitation of the patient? Where are all of these psychotherapists, occupational therapists and social workers going to come from? And how shall *they* be screened for competence?

It is easy to say that psychotherapy or social reform, either one, has fewer immediate risks than surgery or electroshock or radical pharmacotherapy. But there is a problem—and I speak to you now in the most candid way I can. The problem is that whereas the errors of surgeons are soon recognized, the mistakes of psychotherapists and social reformers are less often apparent. This difference is not difficult to understand. Throughout his career a surgeon operates under the constant surveillance of many persons, but it is a rare psychotherapist who retains even a single permanent control. If the social reformer makes a mistake, it may take generations to be recognized, and may well be completely irreversible. Surgeons who often err soon find their referrals drying up; they find themselves shunted into other full-time roles (such as testifying in court), or they restrict their activities to the teaching of medical students, or they go into politics. Perhaps today or tomorrow we will be told where the incompetent social reformer should go. And we would like to know how such a miscreant can be identified, if at all.

Let us suppose that a therapy has a reasonable chance of success and tolerable risks, and that we are confronted with a suitable patient. Then, finally, we may be entitled to offer this procedure to that patient. For a patient to agree in any meaningful way, however, his consent must be "fully informed" (10). But if he has never seen, felt or smelled the complications about which we warn him, how can he be fully informed?

The puzzled patient's usual best recourse is to his own trusted personal physician, the doctor who is on *his* side, who knows *him*, and who has no significant stake in the procedure itself—neither money nor self-esteem nor academic advancement nor scientific achievement. This is surely an important safeguard. But does each of us have a personal physician to whom we can turn for such independent guidance? Do you?

No prisoner has a personal doctor whose allegiance is to him alone. Does this mean that no prisoner should ever have electroshock, behavioral conditioning, or treatment with dangerous drugs? And how about the even more irreversible case of brain surgery? Perhaps with respect to brain surgery at least, we should conclude that prisoners should never have it (11). But what if they want it? Is this not just another infringement on their capacity to choose? Perhaps one solution here would be to say that conviction of a felony carries with it not only the loss of certain civil rights, such as voting or holding office, but also the right to get certain kinds of medical care of the high-risk type. In this way we would inflict an injustice on a few persons in order to safeguard a far greater number. This may seem a workable if not altogether happy solution for prisoners. But how about the fellow who is out on parole and who might actually have access to a personal physician or counselor? Is not the parolee in quite different circumstances than an incarcerated individual?

But none of the above helps us when we are presented with the problem of an individual who has been committed to a mental hospital and can hardly be considered a convicted felon. Nor can he be reasonably considered capable of competent consent. At this juncture, perhaps we can have recourse to some sort of review board, in the Oregon manner. In this case, we keep the individual in custody, hoping he does not meanwhile deteriorate overly much, while five or seven or nine other persons deliberate his fate. Who will pick *them*? Well, on this subject we may have some experience to guide us; and we look forward to hearing about it from Dr. Robert Grimm.

Suppose all other problems are solved, including the patient's informed consent, except that his wife does not consent. Must the next of kin agree? Surely not, you will say, since next of kin are so often of mixed motives anyway. But do not forget that if the patient succumbs, it is the next of kin with whom we must deal. And if the patient does not succumb but merely becomes a complete burden, it is on the next of kin that the burden mainly falls.

Before I close, let me open an altogether different Pandoran box. What if *all* who are directly involved are agreed upon the correct course, but this course has been made illegal by some distant regulatory agency? I have in my own practice two patients whose seizures were apparently well controlled by Elipten; this was withdrawn by the FDA some years ago, and these patients have subsequently never had quite as good control of their seizures. Should I advise them to drive over to Mexico every so often and buy some Elipten there? Most of you here must be aware that many European neurologists consider Tegretol to be one of the very best anticonvulsant medications. Many of us have been recommending it to patients, in spite of the fact that it is not presently (March 1974) FDA approved.

In the state of Massachusetts it is now illegal to give more than thirty-five electroconvulsive treatments to a patient in any calendar year, no matter what the doctor's opinion or the patient's condition. Presumably this number was arrived at by the Massachusetts legislature through some process more responsible than that of the apocryphal state legislature which passed a law that pi equals 3. In any event, to give you only a brief glimpse of what some expect to be the future of medicine, let me quote from a recent article by Alexander (12):

> The capriciousness of temporal law as compared to our own ethics is really grotesque: Two years ago, if a physician performed an abortion he was a criminal, but if subsequently, after his patient developed a severe depression, he brought about her recovery by 40 electroconvulsive treatments, he was a good doctor. Now the situation is reversed: When he performs the abortion he is a good doctor, but if subsequently he finds it necessary to relieve her severe depression by 40 electroconvulsive treatments, he would be a criminal.

Is Dr. Alexander correct when he says that medical morality is superior to temporal law, "just as divine law outranks governmental laws"? Shall we infer from this that we physicians should do what we think is best for our patients, illegal or not, thus deliberately testing bad law with the usual risks of martyrdom in prison?

There are many more questions to be asked, but I should like to end where medical matters are more and more tending to end these days, at least in California. I mean by this, in a civil suit alleging malpractice. What if there is a bad result? If there was a review board, or if the relatives agreed to the course of action, are *all* those who were involved in the decision just as liable as the doctor who actually administered the treatment? How shall recompense be made? Who shall receive the principal recompense? What about the attorney on contingency who risks his time and money organizing an action and may very well end up receiving at least a third of the money awarded for an injury to someone else? Should an attorney receive nothing in spite of his efforts, as often occurs? Can we get some sort of no-fault accident insurance to cover these eventualities? Should relatively desperate remedies be considered the same sort of insurance risks as more standard procedures? As the insurance costs continue to rise astronomically, who will pay for this insurance? And who will profit from its administration?

The experts we are about to hear may give us some answers. Possibly they will give us answers to questions more pressing than the ones which I have raised. Let us recall Gertrude Stein, who when she was about to die asked, "What is the answer?" And receiving none, she uttered her last words, "Well, then, what is the question?"

NOTES

1. Workshop on Psychosurgery, held during the October 1973 meeting in San Diego of the Society for Neuroscience.

2. Sherrington, C. *The Integrative Action of the Nervous System.* Cambridge University Press, 1947.

3. Eccles, J.C. Brain, Speech and Consciousness. *Naturwissenschaften* 60:167-176 (1973).

3a. Nyhan, W.L. Clinical Features of the Lesch-Nyhan Syndrome. *Arch. Int. Med.* 130:186-192 (1972).

4. Chapman, J.S. Peregrinating Problem Patients—Munchausen's Syndrome. *JAMA* 165:927-933, (1957). See also *JAMA* 165:2108; 166:823; 170:843; and 227:799.

5. Smith, W. Lynn, and Philippus, M.J. *Neuropsychological Testing in Organic Brain Dysfunction.* Charles C Thomas, 1969.

6. Lansdell, H. Psychological tests for assessing psychosurgery. *Proc. Amer. Psychol. Assoc.* August 30, 1974.

7. Taub, A., Andy, O.J., and Turnbull, I. Letters to the Editor. *J. Neurosurg.* 40:133-136 (1974).

8. Burgoyne, R. We Contribute to Our Unpopularity. *Bull. So. Calif. Psychoanalytic Soc.* 37:7-9 (1973).

9. Coghill, G.E. The Neuroembryologic Study of Behavior *Science* 78:131-138 (1933).

10. O'Donnell, T.J. Informed Consent. *JAMA* 227:73 (1974).

11. Mark, V.H. and Neville, R. Brain Surgery in Aggressive Epileptics: Social and Ethical Implications. *JAMA* 226:765-772 (1973).

12. Alexander, L. Comments on Presidential Address. *Biol. Psychiat.* 7:193-196 (1973).

*Frontal and Temporal Lobe Lesions and Aggressive Behavior**

ARTHUR KLING
Department of Psychiatry
College of Medicine and Dentistry
of New Jersey-Rutgers Medical School
Piscataway, New Jersey

INTRODUCTION

The role of brain damage as an etiological factor in behavioral disorders must, at this point in time, remain largely speculative. Aside from individual case reports, or in some cases, a small series, there does not exist any significant amount of clinical data on this topic. Some of the major reasons for this lack of data include lack of suitable diagnostic techniques to determine neuropathological changes and their localization. Current diagnostic instruments tend either to be too gross (neurological examination, pneumoencephalography, arteriography, EMI scan) or, as in the case of EEG, to result in rather poor and often paradoxical results when attempts are made to correlate them with behavioral disturbances [although this still remains controversial (1-4)]. Neuropsychological testing is, in a sense, too sensitive, with evidence of minimal and gross dysfunction appearing in such large numbers as to be nondiscriminatory. The same may be

*This research was supported in part by the Behavioral Science Foundation and the Harry B. Frank Guggenheim Foundation.

said of using more refined clinical neurophysiological examinations such as evoked potentials and CNV (Contingent Negative Variation), although these techniques have been applied largely to subjects with minimal brain damage syndrome and to children with perceptual disorders. Even if the techniques currently available were to be applied in a shotgun approach to a large population of behavior disorders, my guess would be that it would result in our finding that most subjects obtained from correctional and court referrals would have a low-to-borderline I.Q.; would show evidence of reading disability and other symptoms related to cognitive-perceptual dysfunction; would also show a high frequency of emotional disturbance and a somewhat higher frequency of nonspecific EEG abnormalities but probably no higher incidence of brain diseases or demonstrable brain pathology than in the nondyssocial population.

While Mark and Ervin (5) have argued that brain dysfunction, particularly that related to temporal lobe disease, may be etiologically significant in aggressive behavior disorders, there is as yet no hard data from well-controlled studies linking specific brain disease to behavioral disorders except with respect to some individual clinical cases with seizure disorders.

This is not to deny or imply that brain dysfunction is not a significant variable in dyssocial behavior. What it means is that we do not yet know the appropriate question to ask of the nervous system or which behavioral variables can best be linked to what neurophysiological variables. Another major problem is that most studies of dyssocial behavior have neglected the ethological or social interactive aspect of human behavior. Little attention has been given to the details of communicative gestures, to the study of individuals in natural or semi-natural settings where social-environmental stimuli resulting in dyssocial behavior occurs. We have put a great deal of emphasis on the sensory-motor-perceptual-cognitive aspects of brain dysfunction, but hardly any at all on the social-behavioral-environmental level.

Serious problems in design methodology and ethical considerations have undoubtedly limited the development of experimental work on human subjects. While progress will be made on neurodiagnosis, clinical neurophysiology and neuropsychology, concurrent animal experimentation may provide some of the appropriate questions, if not answers, to this major social problem.

Field studies of primate social behavior have demonstrated that agonistic behaviors are ubiquitous in primate species and play an essential role in maintaining the integrity of the band and assuring its survival. Intragroup agonism, especially among the males, contributes to the survival and passage of genes which have proven to be successful in maintaining the band as a successful unit. The females, bonded together by familial relationships, also demonstrate hierarchical dominance relationships between themselves, as well as with males in the band. These genealogical relations provide a continuity within the band from one generation to another.

The priority of access to food, space and sex granted to the dominant members of the troop is apparently sufficient reason for subordinate members to strive for higher rank. In most instances, such attempts are composed primarily of nonphysical communications; utilizing vocal, facial and postural signals, either alone or in coalitions with other group members. At times, however, such confrontations may involve physical combat. Direct physical aggression is more common, however, in intergroup or interspecies disputes than among members of the same band.

Because of its complex and multi-determined nature, con-specific aggression is a difficult behavior to discuss, apart from its relationship to environmental, ontogenetic and sexual factors interacting with the nature of the social bondings existing between members of the species.

In the past several decades, a great deal of experimental evidence has been gathered on the identification and manipulation of brain regions involved in the regulation of aggressive behavior. For the past seven years or so, experiments in our laboratory have been utilizing primate social behavior as a model for investigating the neural-hormonal regulation of aggressive and other behaviors central to the maintenance of social bonds in various primate species, including man. In these experiments, we have found that environmental factors, as well as the sex and age of the experimental subjects, are crucial to the expression as well as the sparing of deficits related to the ablation of localized brain structures.

This paper will review the results of some of these experiments and their implications for pathological behavior in man.

METHOD

The general methodology for studying small social groups in our laboratory involves establishing eight to fourteen feral-born adult and juvenile subjects in an 18′ x 10′ x 12′ wire enclosure. The monkeys are provided with chow and water ad libitum. Two weeks after the group is established, time-based quantitative observations of social interactions are initiated. These include joining, play, grooming, huddling, displacement threats, aggression, social distance, cage positions and sexual behaviors. Both the initiators and receivers of these behaviors are recorded. Usually 100 hours of preoperative behavior are collected over a two-to-three-month period, following which the subjects are separated into individual cages and designated animals are operated. After the operates have recovered, the group is reconstituted and another 100 hours or more are collected. The data is analyzed by statistical methods utilizing computer programs for analysis of variance to account for both changes due to the surgery and changes in group behavior over time.

We have, in a number of studies, subsequently transferred the laboratory group to a half-acre enclosure located at the Caribbean Primate Research Laboratory, Sebana Seca, Puerto Rico, and continued the observations in a more natural and spacious setting. Other studies, using *Cercopithicus aethiops*, have involved larger groups of twenty-five or more in our large enclosure in St. Kitts, Eastern Caribbean. In these spacious corrals, social interactions become more meaningful, especially spatial relationships and direct physical aggression.

In totally free-ranging settings, baseline data is collected by locating and following troops, determining their progressions, identifying individuals and habituating them to the presence of observers. Trapping individuals out of a troop can usually be accomplished with appropriate bait in cage-type traps. Once trapped, the subjects are sedated, transported to a local facility, and operated on; along with controls, the subjects are kept in cages until ready for release back into their own troop or in the vicinity of neighboring groups. If the operated subjects reintegrate within the troop, they can be followed and observed. If, however, they become social isolates, it is generally impossible to locate them.

The Temporal Lobe and Related Structures

Bilateral ablation of the temporal lobe—including the uncus, amygdala and hippocampus—in monkeys is well known to result in a behavioral syndrome, described in detail by Klüver (6) as including: 1) a decrease in belligerence and reduction of fear toward normally fear-inducing objects; 2) hyperorality; 3) visual agnosia; and 4) hypersexuality. This syndrome has by now been reproduced in many species of primates, including man (7).

Since these early experiments, considerable attention has been given to fractionating the temporal lobe structures to elucidate specific structures responsible for the syndrome or its components.

Bilateral ablation of the uncus and amygdaloid nuclei without involvement of the hippocampus or the temporal cortex can reproduce the syndrome but is less intense than with involvement of the entire lobe. Portions of the syndrome can also be produced by lesions of the temporal cortex without involvement of the amygdala or hippocampus, especially the reduction in fear of man and to some extent the hyperorality (8).

With respect to amygdala, it now appears that the basal-lateral group of nuclei are responsible for most of the behavioral changes seen after ablation of the entire nucleus. It is not known to what extent the uncal cortex itself is responsible for some of the behavioral changes seen after gross ablations, but stereotaxic lesions of the amygdala, sparing the uncus, have been effective in reproducing the changes seen after the larger lesion (9).

Studies of subjects within several primate species subjected to lesions of the amygdaloid nuclei have now been conducted in artificially composed social groups housed in laboratory enclosures, as well as in semi- and totally natural free-ranging social groups in their natural habitats.

Despite variation in effect due to species-specific behaviors, differing environments and compositions of groups, a number of common features with respect to their social interactions have emerged, which can be summarized as follows: 1) When they are confined and unable to leave the group, lesioned subjects tend to fall in status from previously held positions within the hierarchy. When interacting with one another, lesioned subjects do not seem to have clear dominance relations between them. 2) There is a reduction in positive social behavioral interactions such as joining others, grooming and remaining together. This withdrawal from social interactions may vary from a quantitative reduction in confined settings to total social isolation in the free-ranging condition. In *C. aethiops*, operates withdrew despite attempts by normal group members to interact with them (10). 3) There is a reduction in initiated agonistic behaviors such as threat, aggression and displacement, but this is variable depending greatly on the setting and species. Concomitantly, lesioned subjects tend to respond to aggression by others with fear and withdrawal. In some cases, we have noted a paradoxical increase in aggression, especially in adult females. 4) In general, then, lesions of the amygdaloid nuclei result in a shattering of social bondings, even the mother-infant bonds; further, the social isolation does not tend to diminish over time but may in fact become more intense (3). 5) Despite these deficits seen in social-affective behavior, amygdala-lesioned subjects seem to retain the ability to recognize and respond appropriately to many situations. Reports on human subjects sustaining bilateral amygdalotomy indicate that while affective changes may be considerable, there is a retention of cognitive ability (14). 6) Some symptoms (e.g. hyperorality, hypersexuality) commonly seen in amygdala lesions in laboratory-housed subjects tend to be absent when these subjects are observed in large enclosures or in free-ranging settings. However, in a recent, as yet unpublished, study by Steklis, the Klüver-Bucy syndrome was reproduced in an African green monkey housed in a large outdoor enclosure. This juvenile male, subjected to a large temporal lobe lesion, consistently displayed the hypersexuality, hyperorality and a tendency to approach and explore strange species (donkey, chicken, etc.). Unlike lesions restricted to the amygdala, monkeys with total lobectomy may then display the syndrome in more environmentally complex and social settings.

HUMAN STUDIES

By now there have been a number of patients who have been subjected to either bilateral amygdalectomy (or -otomy) or more extensive temporal lobectomy. These procedures have been carried out largely on temporal lobe epileptics or chronic schizophrenics with or without mental retardation.

A comparison of the results of human studies with those in non-human primates presents certain difficulties in view of the pre-operative neuropsychopathology existing in these cases and in evaluating the effects of the operation in chronically psychotic individuals. Further complications arise when we consider the variability of environments and cultural determinants on human behavior.

A further problem in relating the human and animal studies is that the results of surgical intervention were largely directed to the alleviation of the neuropsychological pathology rather than to detailed behavioral studies of social interactions.

Scoville et al. (11) reported that of five cases of bilateral uncatomy, three showed a decrease of social interaction and decreased aggressiveness. Four out of seven cases of more extensive bilateral medical temporal lobectomy were also less social.

Narabayashi (12) has emphasized that bilateral amygdalotomy, in a large series of hyperactive and aggressive children, may be useful in reducing both symptoms resulting from a variety of congenital brain disorders. Retarded epileptic children became more accessible to training and may be managed outside of institutions. There is an increase in attention span, a decrease in uncontrollable behavior, and in epileptic children, a decrease in clinical seizures. No specific studies were done on social interactions.

Other reports detailing the effects of amygdaloid or temporal lobe lesions in cases of temporal lobe epilepsy generally, but not always, indicate a reduction in episodic violent or disruptive behavior (13).

Gloor (13), on the basis of extensive observations on temporal lobe epileptics, proposed that the higher visual, auditory memory and language function are located in the temporal lobe. It is this brain area that the matching of past and experience takes place, which then activates the anatomically related limbic structures to provide the emotional and motivational significance to this process. The activity of limbic structures, especially the amygdala, then modulates the activity of diencephalic structures, which are responsible for fundamental drive states, including aggressive behavior.

Mark and Ervin (5) have proposed that solid medical evidence exists to link aggressive behavior to focal brain disease. They point out that abnormal aggressiveness is often present in temporal lobe epilepsy, temporal lobe tumors, encephalitis and post-traumatic syndromes.

While the data does not yet exist to substantiate or disclaim these statements except for relatively small members of clinical examples, the largest percentage of persons exhibiting repetitive acts of assaultive or violent behavior probably do not exhibit evidence of gross neurological disease. This is not to suggest that more subtle dysfunction not demonstrable by usual examination procedures may be associated with a larger percentage of violent acts, especially in conjunction with alcohol intoxication. Examination of events surrounding interpersonal crimes of violence frequently implicate alcohol as a contributing factor.

Lesions of Frontal Lobe

Investigations of frontal lobe dysfunction in nonhuman primates have, with some exceptions, focused on fractionating the well-established deficits in delayed response, delayed alternation, conditioning and "drive" inhibition. Hyperactivity, circling and affective changes toward belligerence are regularly found after lobectomy or lesions of the lateral surface. Involvement of the orbital surface may induce apathy, nondirected wandering and discrimination deficits. Little is known, however, about how these deficits affect the behavior of individuals interacting with conspecifics in laboratory or naturally occurring social groups.

Prefrontal lobectomy was shown by Brody and Rosvold (15) to

disrupt the stability of the social hierarchy in a group of juvenile rhesus. Low-ranking operates were noted to inappropriately grab food or attack higher-ranking subjects. Warden and Galt (16) did not observe disruption of dominance relations but grooming behavior disappeared. Deets et al. (17) found that prefrontal lobectomy resulted in social withdrawals with instances of inappropriate aggression despite the subjects being generally less aggressive.

In our laboratory (18), all subjects in a group of eight male juvenile rhesus were sequentially subjected to bilateral ablation of the dorsolateral frontal cortex. The stability of the social hierarchy was not disrupted and all but the dominant monkey spent as much time with the same monkey as he did preoperatively. Four of the eight subjects showed a marked increase in aggression, yet there was a concomitant decrease in threat behavior. Those behaviors which involved direct physical contact, both agonistic and nonagonistic, showed an increase, while those involving affective display diminished. While all subjects engaged in considerable pace stereotypies, it rarely evoked aggressive responses by those who were clearly annoyed by this behavior. It appeared that the deficit in affective communications necessitated the utilization of physical contact.

In a larger, more naturally composed group of stumptailed macaques, in which five of nine subjects were lesioned, there was an increase in total group aggressive behavior. Three female operates fell in rank following an outbreak of violence in which serious physical aggression was directed toward these operates. No inappropriate upward aggression or disruption of feeding was found in the enclosure study (19).

On Cayo Santiago, Meyers et al. trapped five subjects out of one of a number of free-ranging social groups and subjected them to prefrontal lobectomy. After recovery and release, four of the five went solitary, were attacked and chased by normal group members, and eventually died. The youngest operate, a juvenile, reintegrated within the group. In this experiment, adult subjects with control lesions (pinealectomies, superior temporal gyrus lesions) rejoined their groups (20).

Monkeys subjected to selective ablation of the orbital surface of the frontal lobe generally fall from previously held social rank, but unlike amygdaloid animals, it usually takes several months and generally is the result of repeated challenges involving physical aggression by normal group members. Normally, challenges to dominance are not accompanied by a notable amount of physical aggression, but in groups containing frontally lesioned subjects, severe repetitive bouts of physical aggression are not uncommon (21).

Another feature common to orbital lesioned subjects is purposeless wandering and indifference to aggression going on about them. While no totally free field studies have been conducted as yet on monkeys with orbital lesions, their reduced social interactions—including sexual behavior, social indifference and wandering—would make it reasonable to assume they would become social isolates in a free-ranging setting.

Human Studies

Data obtained from the study of human patients subjected to prefrontal lobotomy or lobectomy is difficult to summarize because of the variations in lesion size, areas included and pre-morbid personality. However, the major impairments include the inability of the affected person to adjust behavior to future contingencies, affective lability, lack of initiative, and inattention. Disturbances in judgment, insight and imagination are frequently present.

According to Hecaen (22), in a study of a large series of patients with frontal lobe tumors, the most frequent symptoms were the indifference to surroundings (27%), bradykinesia (22%) and disorientation (21%). Mood changes of euphoria, intolerance and irritability were observed in 37%. Memory disturbances vary widely and are probably related to the size of the lesion.

While the human data does not support any specific relationship between frontal lobe function and aggressive behavior, these commonly associated deficits might, with appropriate social facilitation, lead to persistent inappropriate behavior patterns in some subjects.

DISCUSSION

The presence of lesioned subjects, especially adults, in a restricted group tends to produce an increase in aggressive interactions among the normal members. In some cases, this may be due to repeated challenges to the operates by subordinates, and subsequent displaced aggression when these challenges are unsuccessful. When outbreaks of inappropriate aggression occur, such as within the group of stump-tailed macaques with five dorsolateral lesioned subjects, severe physical injury may occur. It appears that the operates do not exhibit appropriate submissive gestures when threatened and also do not respond to the submissive gestures of the threatened subjects and repeatedly attack them. On the free-ranging rhesus colony of Cayo Santiago, adult frontal lobectomized subjects were repeatedly attacked and some driven into the sea, especially when they wandered into a strange group. Juvenile operates tended to resocialize.

In contrast to groups containing frontal cortex lesioned subjects, those groups in restricted settings with amygdala subjects tend to show reduced levels of agonism when the operates have originated within the group. Their tendency to social indifference and withdrawal does not tend to evoke aggressive attacks by others. In a few cases where we have seen increased aggression, it tends to be more severe and more inappropriately directed than between normal subjects.

I have previously suggested that the social withdrawal characteristic of amygdala-lesioned subjects is related to a disturbance in visual function, in that the more varied and complex the environment, the greater the social withdrawal and the less of the classical syndrome is evident. Horel and Misantane (23) have demonstrated that removing the visual input from striate and pre-striate cortex into the temporal lobe can result in a syndrome closely resembling Klüver and Bucy's original description of temporal lobectomized monkeys. The visual disturbance may be an inability of the lesioned subjects to "sort out" visual information rather than a simple discrimination disability. In addition, disruption of anatomical connections between amygdala and orbital cortex via the medial dorsal thalamic nucleus may contribute to the affective flattening exhibited by monkeys with both amygdala and orbital cortex lesions.

The behavior of monkeys with orbital frontal cortex lesions share additional features with amygdala-lesioned subjects, including the reduction in aggressive behavior, fall in dominance and reduced initiation of social interactions. These changes may also be related to connections between orbital cortex, hypothalamus and dorsal-medial thalamus.

The predominant behavioral changes noted after ablations of the dorsolateral frontal cortex was the increases in aggression, as well as other physical modes of interaction, and reduction of facial and postural gestures. There is still some question of whether these subjects maintain preoperative dominance relations. Where we have seen alterations in social rank, it has been accompanied by serious physical violence. These results imply that the behavioral changes seen after dorsolateral frontal lesions differ significantly from either orbital cortex or temporal lobe ablations. These differences may be related to the more recent evolution and different thalamic projection system of dorsolateral cortex. While there is clearly an affective component to the behavioral syndrome, there appears to be a greater retention of social bondings.

Field studies on naturally composed groups in several species will be necessary before more definite conclusions can be reached regarding the influence of frontal lobe ablations on social-affective behavior.

As has been indicated, it is at present difficult to relate the human and animal lesion effects despite, in some cases, similar brain ablations, not only because of the preexisting neuropsychological pathology in the human reports, but also because the human studies have not focused on social behavior as such. Nevertheless, it would seem possible at this time to design experiments which would come close to the human condition and to conversely study human subjects with social-environmental factors in mind.

NOTES

1. Stevens, J.R. Psychiatric implications of psychomotor epilepsy. *Arch. Gen. Psychiat.* *14*:461-477 (1966).

2. Robbins, E. Antisocial and dyssocial personality disorders. In *Comprehensive Textbook of Psychiatry.* Alfred M. Freedman and Harold I. Kaplan, eds. William Wilkins, Baltimore, 1967.

3. Gibbs, F.A. Clinical correlates of 14 and 6 per record positive spikes. *EEG Clin. Neurophysiol.* *8*:149 (1956).

4. Loomis, S.D. EEG abnormalities as a correlate of behaviors in adolescent male delinquents. *Amer. J. Psychiat.* *125*:12 (1969).

5. Mark, V.H., and Ervin, F.R. *Violence and the Brain.* Harper Row, New York, 1970.

6. Klüver, H. Brain mechanisms and behavior with special reference to the rhiencephalon. *Lancet* 72:567 (1952).

7. Kling, A. Effects of amygdalectomy on social affective behavior in non-human primates. In *The Neurobiology of the Amygdala.* B.E. Eleftheriou, ed. Plenum Publishing Corp., New York, 1972.

8. Akert, K.; Gruesen, R.A.; Woolsey, C.N. and Meyer, D.R. Kluever-Bucy syndrome in monkeys with neocortical ablations of temporal lobe. *Brain* *84*:480-498 (1961).

9. Dryer, T. Behavioral changes following localized lesions of amygdaloid nuclei in the monkey *M. mulatta.* M.S. thesis, University of Illinois, 1972.

10. Kling, A.; Lancaster, J., and Benitone, J. Amygdalectomy in the free-ranging vervet. *J. Psychiat. Res.* 7:191 (1970).

11. Scoville, W.B.; Dunsmore, R.H.; Liberson, W.T.; Henry, C.E. and Pepe, A. Observations on medial temporal lobotomy uncotomy in the treatment of psychotic states. Proceedings of the Association on Research on Nervous and Mental Disease 31, 347, 1953.

12. Narabayashi, H. Stereotaxic amygdalotomy. In *The Neurobiology of the Amygdala.* B.E. Eleftheriou, ed. Plenum Publishing, New York, 1972.

13. Gloor, P. Temporal lobe epilepsy. In *The Neurobiology of the Amygdala.* B.E. Eleftheriou, ed. Plenum Publishing Corp., New York, 1972.

14. Anderson, R. Psychological difference after amygdalectomy. *Acta Neurologica Scand. Suppl.* *43*:46-94 (1970).

15. Brody, E.B., and Rosvold, H.E. Influence of prefrontal lobotomy on social interaction in a monkey group. *Psychosom. Med.* *14*:406-415 (1952).

16. Warden, C.J., and Galt, W. A study of cooperation, dominance, grooming and other social factors in monkeys. *J. Genet. Psychol.* *63*:213-233 (1943).

17. Deets, A.C.; Harlow, H.F.; Singh, S.D. and Bloomquist, A.J. Effects of bilateral lesions of the frontal granular cortex on the social behavior of rhesus monkeys. *J. Comp. Physiol. Psychol.* 72:452-461 (1970).

18. Miller, M.H., and Kling, A. Social behavior in a confined group of juvenile macaques sustaining dorsolateral frontal lesions. 5th Congress of Internat. Primatol. Soc., Nagoya, Japan, August 1974.

19. Mass, R. The effects of dorsolateral frontal ablations on the social behavior of a caged group of eleven stumptail macaques. *Primates*: in press.

20. Meyers, R.; Miller, M.H. and Swett, C. Changes in social affinity following pre-frontal and cingulate lesions in free-ranging macaques. *Brain Res. 64*:257-269 (1973).

21. Notkin, E. Effects of orbital lesions on the social behavior of the caged stumptailed macaque (*Macaca speciosa*). M.S. thesis, Rutgers University, 1972.

22. Hecaen, H. Mental symptoms associated with tumors of the frontal lobe. In *The Frontal Granular Cortex and Behavior.* J. Warren and K. Akert, eds. McGraw-Hill, New York, 1964.

23. Horel, J.A., and Misantane, L.J. The Kluever-Bucy syndrome produced by partial isolation of the temporal lobe. *Exp. Neurol.* 42:101-112 (1974).

Evaluation of Organic Factors in Patients with Impulse Disorders and Episodic Violence

FRANK R. ERVIN
Department of Psychiatry
School of Medicine
University of California
Los Angeles, California

I would like to say hurriedly and somewhat defensively that I'm not a surgeon, and I don't believe in applying psychosurgery to violent individuals; in fact, I fought vigorously for some years against the notion of enforced therapy of prisoners. But I definitely would like to tell you about the development and history of my own interest in prison populations. I think this will bring out some problems that are relevant to the topic to this symposium.

As most of you do know, since about 1952, I've been interested in the problem of temporal lobe epilepsy, and particularly in the behavior disorders associated with it; in fact, I can claim to have some small experience in that interesting syndrome, which Hughlings Jackson described around the turn of the century as the key to understanding insanity. He recognized early, as I was later to be persuaded is true, the existence of an intermittent pathological syndrome in man which is related to a definable structural and, in principle, physiological brain dysfunction; at one time or another, this syndrome replicated, in a wide spectrum of patients, all of the psychopathological phenomena which psychiatrists are accustomed to dealing with in full psychiatric cases, and it provides an unusual experimental model for the understanding of some psychiatric disorders.

While I was at Harvard, the opportunity arose to work with Drs. William Sweet and Vernon Mark, who had for the previous fifteen years been involved in trying to refine neurosurgical procedures; they had a particular interest, though not a central one, in temporal lobe epilepsy and its surgical treatment. The collaboration turned out to be extraordinarily fruitful for all of us as we attempted to gain an understanding of some of the temporal lobe mechanisms in man. As you perhaps know—and there is some controversy surrounding both the data and the interpretations thereof—we felt that we could generalize as follows from our experiences with some twenty patients we had looked at who had been operated upon for their intractable temporal lobe epilepsy: in those that had a concomitant disorder of impulse control, characterized by intermittent attack behavior, we could indeed find some correlations between the activity and dysfunction of certain brain structures, specifically in the amygadala region, and the appearance of this unique intermittent behavioral disorder. Now, thinking about those patients and that problem and assuming (as we did) that it was reasonable to think that there are some individuals who have a focal brain abnormality in the temporal lobe which is related (though multifactorally, in a causal rather than casual way) to the appearance of episodic attack behavior, then we found it only logical to add that if we were to look at individuals characterized by recurrent attack behavior, even if we were not necessarily presented with other intermittent traditional symptoms of temporal lobe disease (i.e. neurological fits), we might also find that those individuals had a similar or related disturbance of temporal lobe or amygdaloid mechanism. Now, that logic led us to do something that usually doesn't work around a hospital: I simply phoned our walk-in emergency psychiatric clinic and said, "Listen, if you ever see anybody who presents a chief complaint of recurrent attack behavior, I'd like to have a look at him. Would you send him up?" Busy residents rarely remember such requests, but in fact, we started getting two to three referrals a day from our own outpatient clinic. Soon people were coming in from all over town, and not too long after that, they were hiking halfway across the country; people with duffel bags were turning up in the front office and saying, "I just came in from Illinois, and here's my problem!"

Since that time I have seen or communicated with some three or four hundred such patients, some in consultation, some via letters and telephone calls; they exist in large numbers. Having opened that valve, we started doing some obvious things and suddenly realized we had run into a rather intractable problem—namely, that our hypothesis clearly was focal temporal lobe damage, that's what we wanted to look for, and yet we had no tools to do so. In fact, as one runs through the diagnostic armamentarium of the neurologist or psychiatrist, those procedures designed specifically to investigate the integrity of the limbic system functions are quickly countable—i.e., practically nonexistent. However, what we tried to do was use those procedures that seemed reasonable from a traditional point of view; in our work-up we fell back on a more general line of questioning: What are these people like? Do they differ from a general population? Can one in fact suggest that there is anything wrong with neuro-humoral function of the kind that should be causally or even plausibly related to their behavior disorder?

We have already reported on the first 130-odd of those cases, and what was concluded about them was roughly the following: after we had screened out a large number of obviously inappropriate cases—adolescents whose parents brought them in for temper tantrum, the mentally retarded, overt paranoid schizophrenics, obsessives afraid that they might commit violence because they had thought about it a lot—what we had left was a population, half of whom were most parsimoniously accounted for in rather traditional psychiatric terms, such as character disorders or mixed neuroses, borderline states of one kind or another. In general, historically, although members of this group often had histories of large numbers of assaults or attacks on other people, these were by and large very narrowly and specifically defined cases of aggression. For example, every time his mother-in-law came over, the son-in-law would get into a fight with her; sometimes he would knock her down, and sometimes he would break a rib, but on no other occasions was he in trouble. Although people such as this form a very interesting population, an important one for any overall consideration of the problem of violent behavior in our society, and so on, I was not especially interested in these people. For our research purposes, we defined violent behavior as the physical attack of one person upon another with whom he was in face-to-face confrontation, which if carried out would lead to physical injury, or indeed death. For practical purposes, as we began to define a specific study population, we asked for at least three such events in the previous two years, and a witness to them; we would not take a self-referred patient's word that he had in fact carried out these acts, because people do lie about their behavior.

After having screened out obviously inappropriate cases and conventional psychiatric ones, the population we were left with was of particular interest; roughly half of this group demonstrated what we felt was suggestive evidence of brain disorder—most commonly temporal lobe disorder. This conclusion was based on relatively weak clinical findings, focal EEG abnormalities. If other symptomatology justified it, further tests were ordered, with pneumoencephalographs sometimes showing evidence of dilated temporal horns asymmetrically; occasionally brain scan evidence, and interestingly, a large number of impairments of asymmetry of coordination, some speech difficulties, perhaps a small eye field, asymmetrical vestibular dysfunctions, and so on—no overwhelmingly strong evidence, to be sure.

Let me describe the model patient in the other half of the group—that is to say, patients in whom one could define nothing objective that was suggestive of focal brain disease, but whose clinical history was very similar to the histories of those with brain disorders. He is male, ten to one over females in our experience (national violent crime figures are five to one over female); he made his first violent attack—in terms of personal assault—sometime shortly after puberty, almost never before; prior to puberty he was consistently recognized as a "problem child," even to himself; he was a chronic runaway; he was a late bed-wetter; he was prone to temper tantrums; he had a reasonably high incidence of being noted by teachers or parents to be cruel to animals; fire setting was a very common childhood problem, the one that has most commonly brought him to the attention of the authorities (not physical attack until post-puberty, by and large). After puberty he had a peculiar, and to use an old term, polymorphous perverse sexual adjustment. He is considered to be a restless, trouble-making, short-attention-span individual; he is impulsive in many regards. He usually finds himself a niche in the economic world that does not have to make him too settled, such as a truckdriving, construction work, the merchant marine, something of that kind.

The people we were seeing were mostly white males at a private, rather high-class hospital in Boston, so they were preselected by region; these were people who bring themselves to such a private hospital, so by and large they were working, could hold down jobs. Sixty percent of this group had had at least one arrest and conviction for a crime of personal violence. So they had been defined at least once by the social system as being "criminal." Indeed, of the eight murderers in this one hundred and thirty people, three were by self-report multi-murderers (at least to us); most of them had records to back it up and had gotten off on such charges as manslaughter or justifiable homicide. One, for instance, walked in and said, "You've got to do something to help me. I've literally this minute walked out of the grand jury hearing which cleared me of the murder of a close friend of mine. But I did it, it *was* a murder; I've nearly done it before and I know I'll do it again unless you can do something to help me." Their violent acts were in no way the trivial breaking of teacups on the back porch.

In giving the background of their attack behavior, they sometimes mention that acts of violence were characteristically presaged by some prodromal state which they could often identify. Interestingly enough, this information is rarely volunteered. I only stumbled onto this fairly late: after our group or I had been seeing someone for a while, he would eventually come in one day and say something like, "Well, this is one of those weeks when it blew and I'm in trouble. "(What happened?)" "Well, I got up in the morning and I had that feeling I always have when things are going to go bad." "(Oh, really, why don't you tell us about that feeling you always have.)" "Vague, though in the general area . . . butterflies in my stomach, a tight band around my head, flashing lights in the left visual field—" A wife might chime in: "Yah, he always looks kinda funny. I think his mouth droops a little bit on days like that. I always know when he's going to do it." "(What do you do when you feel like that?) Usually he mentions one of two things: either he does nothing—he goes on about his business—or he tries to self-medicate. In general he uses alcohol for self-medication, of these people, and by general report of these people, the drinking of alcohol does not improve the situation. Indeed, it usually makes the dysphoric internal state worse and contributes, I think, to a greater loss of control when the trigger comes along. Such a dysphoric state might last as long as two or three days.

During the course of the next hours or days, some trigger of face validity would occur—that is to say, a provocation would arise, perhaps some small event which, looked at from the outside is barely understandable as a provocation. A classic example is provided by a fellow who finally got to me because his mistress brought him in while his wife was in the hospital as a result of the following sequence of events: Morning scene at the breakfast table. He says, "Do we have to have burnt toast for breakfast every morning?" She says, "If you don't like the way the toast is fixed, why don't you make your *own* goddamned toast?" Shortly after that, an ambulance was called to take her to the hospital with a fractured mandible, a fractured clavicle, three fractured ribs, and a ruptured spleen that had to be surgically removed. He came in led by someone else, full of remorse, depressed; he was weeping, and pointed out that he had done this several times in the preceding two years, once nearly killing his child; he seemed very upset about his behavior, reporting, as nearly half of this group did, previous suicidal gestures while in the depths of despair over their behavior and the consequences to the world around them.

Another such case: this man finally said to me, "I have this feeling . . . " and began to describe it. What he did was go to work (he was a machinist); he had been there about an hour when his buddy walked up behind him, unseen, slapped him on the back, and said, "Hey, you old m. f., how are you today?" This man turned around and clubbed his friend with the wrench he had in his hand. I asked, "Well, then how did you feel?" "I felt a lot better," he replied. He went home and then became extremely depressed. I emphasize this depression because it is fairly common and often quite intense. In his case it led (as it does in many) to going to sleep, and then waking up, feeling pretty good internally, but feeling quite remorseful and upset about what had happened. After this man got up, he went to his friend's house, apologized to him and his wife, and then came in the next day quite upset about what had happened.

With these people there is a fairly consistent pattern of pathological aggression; these are as a rule rather passive and ineffectual, generally dependent, and somewhat infantile men, if I can speak in those terms, who perhaps with some rising tension eventually respond to some particular trigger, but always overreact. They are quite different from the character disorder group, many of whom carry a very high level of tension all the time and then some particular input pushes them over their threshold.

The frequency of these episodes in most of the group we looked at range from something like four to twenty per year; many of them have rather significant episodes as frequently as once a week, though not necessarily sending someone to the hospital in each case. Another, although not common, characteristic is a redirection of attack behavior toward themselves which shows up sometimes in the absence of a target. A case in point would be the man who beat his wife almost regularly, once a week or so. One evening the wife locked herself in the bathroom; because he couldn't break down the door, he stood in front of it shouting at his wife, and finally he took off his shoe and beat himself in the face. He had to be carried off to the hospital to have some plastic repair of the face.

Ten percent of the members of this group were afraid to drive, and in fact many had turned in their driver's license. They reported that they were good drivers on the highway, but that in the city, when someone would cut them off on the road, their impulse was to floorboard the car and smash into the other driver. Or they would chase someone that had passed them and drive the other car off the road a mile or so later. They were quite concerned about their driving habits, and again, this impulsive response was quite characteristic.

We tried various methods with these men that I won't report on at great length; we worked with some of them in group or individual therapy, and most were carried on drugs at one time or another. There were various manipulations of their environment: for example, their wives (who were a special subpopulation) were taken into group therapy. As we began to work with them, it became clear to me that the following sequence of events was true.

First, this is a behavioral problem (I was about to say syndrome, but it might not be quite that strong) that is thoroughly neglected in medicine. Eighty percent of these men had sought medical help before they saw us and had essentially been turned away, often turned away repeatedly. In one classic case, the patient had come to the hospital eighteen times, each time only to be diagnosed as a sociopath and to be dismissed. These men had committed themselves to state hospitals, hoping to get treatment and protection from their own impulses. On occasion they had even had themselves locked up by an understanding sheriff or a local police station; they were very concerned about their problem in between attacks.

In trying to figure out why they weren't seen and cared for, I looked at the figures in our Massachusetts General Hospital walk-in psychiatric clinic, which had 15,000 patient-visits a year when I was there a few years ago. Five percent of these were for "violent behavior," and that figure includes paranoids, schizophrenics, alcoholic excitements, and a number of other things; violent behavior is a common presenting complaint to a psychiatric unit. It became clear that these men weren't looked at for two reasons. First, they're scary and unpleasant people. They're very difficult to work with: even though they were all self-referred and highly motivated, if one, for example, had to wait an hour to take a test, he would tend to blow his top and walk out, but he would come back two days later, very remorseful. After being placed on medication, he could go a week without an event, but would then likely say, "I'm not going to take these goddamned pills every day," and would throw them down the toilet. Then following that, he would have some episode and come back in a week. In the first three months of our study, I felt we'd never complete a work-up on any patient because they all disappeared somewhere in the course of it. However, by the time a year had passed, we had regained all our patients. They all kept coming back. They're desperate for help, but they all have this impulsive, ambivalent, paranoid attitude toward it. So they are very difficult, and for the average doctor they are certainly scary and worse to work with in some ways than alcoholics.

Second, these men are not at this point within a traditional framework of a diagnostic strategy or a therapeutic strategy. It is not clear what one can do about them. Their case is similar to that of the person who comes in and says he is possessed. It is very difficult to doctors to go through an orderly diagnostic and therapeutic procedure if we have not been specially trained in that particular area, but I felt that it was terribly important that these people received a work-up. There were some who were likely to turn up with treatable diseases; and indeed, out of this first group, seven had rather classic temporal lobe epilepsy which no one had previously recognized. They were simply turned over to the neurology clinic to be followed and treated. I've also picked up two cases of hypoglycemia and some other traditional medical things. If you look at these cases as a medical problem, you find something that contributes to it. Certainly if one corrects that specific dysfunction, then you no longer see, or you see less frequently, these episodes of assault behavior.

As we amassed more data, we began to really get some notion of the incidence in the community of this kind of thing.

The next idea that occurred to us was that if these men who are bringing themselves in and are so concerned about their behavior have as high an incidence of "criminal history" as they seem to be reporting, then this population overlaps in a nonzero sense with a "criminal justice population." They go to jail, get out, they come to see us and work with us for a while, and then they get arrested again and perhaps get put back in jail, and so on. Doesn't it seem likely that of those people going through the criminal justice system who are now defined as impulsive criminals or violent criminals or what-not, some of them might be part of a group with an identifiable disease? Has anybody ever looked into who's in that system, how did they get there, and what are their characteristics?

I needn't remind you that there is no tradition or law that mandates neuromedical or neurobiological evaluation of anybody appearing before a court of law. In those states where cases of homicide involved an obligatory psychiatric evaluation, that psychiatric evaluation is ordinarily poorly done. Even if it is done well, the issues in question are traditional psychodynamic ones: Is he oriented? Is he schizophrenic? Can he stand trial? The questions are not addressed to the issue of how intact his cerebral function is. There is no such tradition in the law, as I say, so there is nothing known about that level of dysfunction.

We then decided to look at the prison system and at the question of who is in fact in prison. The courts cannot provide information on who floats through there. The prison system turns out to be very interesting historically. It wasn't much over a hundred years ago that in the United States little or no distinction was made between various kinds of dyssocial behavior. People whom we would now call criminal and those we would now call "crazy" and those who were at that time called "paupers" were by and large all locked up together. Eventually a subset of that population was teased out, defined as "crazy," and put into mental hospitals. From then on, at least from the time of Kraepelin, an orderly taxonomy was devised, the usual processes of science were pursued: subgroups were defined, rationales were looked for, treatments were tested out, and indeed, with all the current talk about psychiatry and its limitations, between 1900 and about 1950 many of the major psychiatric problems of the 1900's, such as syphilis, pellagra, and bromism, were cured and moved to other disciplines. The major hospital populations of the mental hospitals at the turn of the century were systematically subdefined, and by and large, treatments and general preventions were delineated, leaving us with an ever-dwindling wastebasket of focal schizophrenics and "seniles." Indeed, there is now some slow whittling into these populations. That process of careful taxonomy, investigation, therapeutic trial, and so on was never carried out on the residual population that was left defined as "criminal," and that, I think, was for three reasons: First was the overly repressive moralism of a Calvinist society. Second, the misapplication of naive and mechanistic late-nineteenth-century biology led to a kind of Lombroso type of phenomenon, simple-minded explanations of different types of murder and so on which generally didn't work and were both intellectually and ethically reprehensible to many people. Third, at about that time, with the failure of traditional biology in the area, the emerging science of sociology came on the scene and began to make some sense out of those populations. That is, sociologists could now come in, look at the prison population, and say who was there, and on the demographic level it turns out not to have changed that much even today. At the turn of the century, the people who got into jail were the poor, the fatherless boys, urban displaced persons, and so on. I won't take you through all the criminal statistics, but we began to get some orderly descriptions of those populations on the sociological, and later on the individual psychological, scale, and these descriptions began to be used as causal explanations. If who's in prison is poor, then if one gets rid of poverty, there would be fewer people in prison—a *non sequitur*, but both ethically and morally appealing, and anybody who's interested in human beings would like to wipe out poverty anyway. So that was as good an explanation as any. However, since 1888 nobody has gone through the prison and done a systematic biomedical examination of every man in that prison; in fact, that is what we proposed to undertake. We haven't done that adequately by any manner of means, so I don't have a lot of data to report, but to make the point with two or three things that have come out of the data, we found that it's one thing to be violent on the street, and it is quite another to lose control of your impulses in the presence of the guards and other prisoners. Looking at who is violent within the prison, we wound up with an excruciatingly matched population, in I.Q.'s, nature of committing crimes and so on. The following was found true: for the prison population as a whole, there is a high level of violent acts immediately after admission and for about three weeks. Then it drops and becomes quite stable and rises only just before parole board hearings, which is an interesting separate phenomenon. I think it is more sociopsychological. There is, however, in the prison a group whose level of violent acts is like that of the men in the hospital study mentioned earlier. If you take these two groups, compare them, and look back in time as to who they are, this group is the one that has a history of recurrent acts of violence on the street, drawn from probation, parole, and self-reported records. Now that fits with all the courts' statistics that "crimes of personal violence" tend to be self-repeated. The President's commission analysis, phrased in an awkward way, is that of all those people standing before the bar accused of crimes of personal violence, 85 percent have been there before. The single biggest longitudinal study is that of Wolfgang in Philadelphia, with a cohort of 15,000 youths followed from age twelve; of those who committed recurrent delinquent acts (nearly everybody committed one; that is part of growing up, one of Wolfgang's points) six percent of them accounted for 64 percent of all the crimes of personal violence. There is therefore a small subpopulation even within the criminal population, and I suggest that they deserve to be looked at.

REFERENCES

Wolfgang, M.E. *Crime and Race: Conceptions and Misconceptions.* New York: Institute of Human Relations Press, 1964.

Wolfgang, M.E. *Patterns in Criminal Homicide.* Philadelphia, University of Pennsylvania Press, 1958.

Brain Stimulation and the Origin of Violent Behavior

ELLIOT S. VALENSTEIN
Department of Psychology and Neuroscience Laboratory
University of Michigan
Ann Arbor, Michigan

Thomas Hobbes described the life of man in his natural state as "solitary, poor, nasty, brutish, and short." Generalizing from the fiercely competitive society in which he lived, he concluded that without civilization, "war of every man against every man" would be the rule. A century later, after explorers had returned with descriptions of life in Samoa, Tahiti, and Hawaii, it was possible to speak of the "noble savage" and the inherent goodness of man. Today, few people attach much significance to questions about the basic nature of man, as ethnologists have made it clear that, depending upon their social and physical environments, humans exhibit great differences in behavior. The point is well illustrated in Colin Turnbull's (1972) account of the transformation of the Ik, an African people forced to change from a life of successful hunting to that of farming under the most difficult of circumstances. Within three generations their social organization had deteriorated and the struggle for individual survival made them hostile and as "generally mean as any people could be." This is the perspective that must be maintained above all else when we try to understand the increases in violent behavior presently going on in our society.

It is not necessary to accept Locke's view of man at birth as a tabula rasa in order to stress the paramount role of environmental factors. There may very well be some universal motor patterns of attack and defense that reflect the organization of the nervous system. There may also be some universal stimulus situations that are likely to evoke these motor patterns, as Eibl-Eibesfeldt (1974) has argued. It is obvious, however, that these "universals" of human nature cannot account for the wide differences in overt violent behavior that exist between peoples and at different periods among the same people.

Although there is every reason to believe that the present increase in violence is related to changes in the conditions of our lives, it is difficult to find agreement on the main causes of the problem or the remedies that should be implemented. Understandably, we are anxious about the dangers, angry at the senseless killings, and perhaps most of all frustrated over our inability to stop the trend. In the face of this frustration, it is not completely surprising that biological proposals have found a receptive audience. After all, we have to do something! Biological solutions have even gained support where one would least expect to find it, among social scientists. In his Presidential Address to the American Psychological Association, Kenneth Clark, a social psychologist, startled many in his audience by remarking that

> given the urgency of the immediate survival problem, the psychological and social sciences must enable us to control the animalistic, barbaric and primitive propensities in man and subordinate these negatives to the uniquely human moral and ethical characteristics of love, kindness and empathy. We can no longer afford to rely solely on the traditional prescientific attempts to contain human cruelty and destructiveness.
>
> Given these contemporary facts, it would seem that a requirement imposed on all power-controlling leaders, and those who aspire to such leadership, would be that they accept and use the earliest perfected form of psychotechnological, biochemical intervention which would assure their positive use of power and reduce or block the possibility of using power destructively. (Clark, Presidential Address, American Psychological Association, 1971)

Clark, as a social scientist, does not recommend any specific biological intervention, but Vernon Mark and Frank Ervin (1970) are in a position to be much more specific in their recommendations. Mark and Ervin, respectively, a neurosurgeon and neuropsychiatrist, have stressed the magnitude of the problem of violence in the United States and strongly suggest that biological interventions can make a significant contribution toward a solution. Although their book, *Violence and the Brain*, contains perfunctory concessions to environmental factors, these are more than counterbalanced by statements criticizing (often unfairly) the inability of such factors to explain the occurrence of violence. Recently, while denying any racial ramifications of a biological emphasis, Mark (1974) continues to de-emphasize the importance of environmental factors:

> It is our experience that there is no special correlation between violence and race. The physician in the emergency room and the clinic witness the results of violence in both upper class and lower class homes. Although ghetto violence may be reported more often and may be more visible due to its spilling out of overcrowded homes into the streets, from the physician's perspective the color of violence is claret, not black or white.
>
> The victims of unreported violence are just as severely injured as the ghetto victims of blunt instruments or knives . . . The disproportionate prevalence of violence in the ghetto becomes more apparent than real in light of . . . widespread automobile violence and the domestic violence that is more often revealed in the divorce court than in the police court. (Mark, 1974, pp. 224-225)

If one believes that people of all walks of life are equally inclined to violence (in spite of overwhelming evidence to the contrary), environmentally oriented solutions are very likely to be perceived as ineffective. Thus Mark and Ervin write:

> One might summarize the sociological approaches by saying that social disintegration, frustrations and aggressions, and the subcultural norms of violence all play a part in generating violent behavior. There seems, however, to be no general agreement among sociologists or cultural anthropologists on the relative importance of these mechanisms; nor have these theories led, as yet, to definitive programs which have reduced the incidence of the violent behavior in our society. (Mark and Ervin, 1970, p. 150)

If environmental factors have been exaggerated, or at least if environmentally oriented programs are destined to be ineffective, then biological solutions gain in attractiveness. The preface to *Violence and the Brain* begins: "We have written this book to stimulate a new and biologically oriented approach to the problem of human violence" (Mark and Ervin, 1970, Preface). The extent of the problem is indicated shortly afterwards:

> Violence is, without question, both prominent and prevalent in American life. In 1968 more Americans were the victims of murder and aggravated assault in the United States than were killed and wounded in seven-and-one-half years of the Vietnam War; and altogether almost half a million of us were the victims of homicide, rape, and assault. (Mark and Ervin, 1970, p. 3)

The impression that brain abnormalities may contribute substantially to this massive problem is conveyed early in the book: "Most people consider brain disease to be a rare phenomenon. It is likely, however, that more than ten million Americans suffer from an obvious brain disease, and the brains of another five million have been subtly damaged." (Mark and Ervin, 1970, p. 5)

Because the statistics on the incidence of brain abnormalities are so intimately coupled to descriptions of violent crimes, only very critical readers of *Violence and the Brain* will fail to draw the conclusion that there is a causal relationship. It might not be irrelevant in this context to mention Michael Crichton's novel, *The Terminal Man.* It is generally recognized that this book was influenced in a number of obvious ways by Mark and Ervin's thesis and case descriptions. At one point in the novel, Ellis, a neurosurgeon, explains on television the rationale for implanting electrodes in the brain of a patient:

> "The patient," Ellis answered, "suffers from intermittent attacks of violent behavior. He has organic brain disease—his brain is damaged. We are trying to fix that. We are trying to prevent violence."
>
> No one could argue with that, he thought. . . .
>
> "Is that common, brain damage associated with violence?"
>
> "We don't know how common it is," Ellis said. "We don't even know how common brain damage alone is. But our best estimates are that ten million Americans have obvious damage, and five million more have a subtle form of it."
>
> "Fifteen million?" one reporter said. "That's one person in thirteen." . . .
>
> "Something like that," he replied on the screen. "There are three quarters of a million people with cerebral palsy. There are over four million with convulsive disorders, including epilepsy. There are six million with mental retardation. There may be as many as two and a half million with hyperkinetic behavior disorders."
>
> "And all of these people are violent?"
>
> "No, certainly not. But an unusually high proportion of violent people, if you check them, have brain damage. Physical brain damage. Now, that shoots down a lot of theories about poverty and discrimination and social injustice and social disorganization. Those factors contribute to violence, of course. But physical brain damage is also a major factor. And you can't correct physical brain damage with social remedies." . . .
>
> "When you say violence—"
>
> "I mean," Ellis said, "attacks of unprovoked violence initiated by single individuals. It's the biggest problem in the world today, violence. And it's a huge problem in this country. In 1969, more Americans were killed or attacked in this country than have been killed or wounded in all the years of the Vietnam war."

How very closely Ellis' arguments follow those of Mark and Ervin is apparent. Also captured very well in Ellis' comments is the general impatience (if not disdain) with environmental explanations. Particularly revealing is the fact that Crichton, who has a medical degree, was moved to add the following postscript to later printings of his novel: "I am persuaded that the understanding of the relationship between organic brain damage and violent behavior is not so clear as I thought at the time I wrote the book."

Mark and Ervin present the evidence for the belief that there is a strong relationship between violent behavior and convulsive disorders, particularly those associated with temporal lobe disorders. There is no doubt that there is evidence that can be mustered to support this conclusion (for example, see Mark and Sweet, 1974). In some instances of clear brain damage, reparative surgery has been successful in reducing very disruptive violent behavior (Gloor, 1967). To put such evidence in better perspective, it is necessary to emphasize several points. First, there is no convincing evidence that these cases of episodically occurring violence caused by brain pathology represent anything more than a very insignificant percentage of the violence in our society. Certainly there is no reason to believe that brain pathology is contributing to the accelerating rate of assaultive behavior. Secondly, violent behavior has not been observed only after damage to the temporal lobes. Reeves and Plum (1969), for example, have described a case of a woman in which the incidence of rage attacks (as well as other symptoms) could be traced to a medial hypothalamic neoplasm. Other cases, implicating other parts of the brain, could easily be cited. To suggest that a significant amount of violence is due to temporal lobe abnormality is misleading both in its overemphasis of the temporal lobes and in the implication that a substantial part of the total violence in our society can be attributed to brain damage.

The belief that violent behavior and temporal lobe epilepsy are commonly associated has been used to bolster the argument that violence is often the result of brain pathology. Many clinicians, however, refute the claim of a strong relationship between epilepsy and violence. Current estimates of the incidence of violence among epileptics range between 1 and 4 percent. Even some of this "violence" is thought to be an indirect effect of the disorder, occurring when well-meaning people have attempted to restrain an epileptic during a postictal confusional state. Moreover, if allowances are made for age differences (temporal lobe epileptics are older on the average than other epileptics), the incidence of violence is probably not higher for the temporal lobe subgroup. Reports still appear claiming a strong relationship between temporal lobe epilepsy and aggressive behavior, but a recent review of the literature concluded that the relationship has been exaggerated (Goldstein, 1974).

Although the disagreement about violent behavior and temporal lobe epileptics is likely to continue, there seems to be a general consensus that assaultive behavior is unlikely to occur during a seizure. Gloor (1967), who has had an opportunity to observe many temporal lobe seizures at the Montreal Neurological Institute, concluded that "rage, with or without aggressive behavior, is an extremely rare ictal phenomenon." This seems to be equally true of psychomotor epilepsy, in spite of claims to the contrary. Rodin (1973), for example, found no relationship in an experiment in which seizures were induced by administering the EEG-activating drug bemigride. He reported that no incident of violence was seen during or after the psychomotor automatisms induced in 57 epileptic patients.

It is easy to create the impression that temporal lobe brain injuries contribute significantly to the problem of violence by selecting evidence and presenting it in a manner and a context that will maximize the impact. A description of Charles Whitman, the man who committed mass murder from the University of Texas tower, provides a particularly illustrative example:

> Whitman kept voluminous personal diaries, similar in detail to those of President Kennedy's murderer, Oswald. In the last several months of his life Whitman noted in writing that something peculiar was happening to him which he did not understand, but was recording in the hope that its mention would help others to do so. In March of 1966 he consulted one of the University of Texas' psychiatrists, blurting out early in the interview that sometimes he became so mad he could "go up to the top of that University tower and start shooting at people." In mid-August of 1966, after murdering his mother and his wife in their apartments and the female receptionist at the top of the tower, he then stepped out on to the parapet and killed by gunfire 14 people, wounding 24 others. His postmortem examination disclosed the highly malignant type of primary infiltrating tumor of the brain called a glioblastoma multiforme. The substantial damage to the brain from the gunshot wounds which terminated the murderer's barrage led the neuropathologist not to examine it by the standard procedures. Hence he is uncertain as to the precise location of the tumor, but he thinks that the walnut-sized mass was probably in the medial part of one temporal lobe. (Sweet, Ervin and Mark, 1969)

The quotation should be examined critically. Why, for example, is Oswald mentioned since the only connection established with Whitman is that they both kept diaries? Why is it implied that Whitman killed his mother, wife, receptionist and fourteen others all in quick succession? The description certainly is consistent with the impression that the mass murders were committed in the throes of a sudden, episodic attack of violence. Actually, Whitman killed his mother and wife the night before. There was nothing episodic about any of the event. Whitman described his plan in his diary down to the details about the clothing he would wear, the defense of his position on the tower, and plans for an escape. It is also clear that the "evidence" about the location of the brain tumor has been shaped to conform to the bias of the authors. The shotgun damage to the brain and its subsequent mishandling made it impossible to locate the tumor with any certainty. It could not be clearly established that the tumor was in the temporal lobes, let alone the "medial part," where, not too coincidentally, the amygdala resides. Equally revealing are the omissions from the account. There was much in Whitman's childhood background that could have suggested alternative explanations of his mental disturbance and propensity for violence that was never mentioned. It is difficult to establish how much of the total evidence supporting the view of a unique relationship between the temporal lobes and violence is based on this type of evidence, but it is clear that much of the evidence has been filtered by a biased screening process.

Mark and Ervin clearly believe that abnormal brain foci in the amygdala trigger episodes of violence in a greater number of instances than previously suspected. They point out that these "brain triggers" may not be evident during a routine or even an "activated" EEG examination. It is suggested that implanted electrodes may be helpful in locating these abnormal foci because they can be used to monitor electrical activity from deep brain structures and with the aid of telemetering devices continuous recordings can be obtained. The implanted electrodes can also be used to stimulate the brain. It is argued that the initiation of violent outbursts (similar to the patient's "spontaneous" assaultive behavior) by stimulation can reveal the neural foci that normally triggers this behavior. Lastly, if the abnormal brain site is located, a small discrete lesion can eliminate the source of the problem without producing any of the great number of undesirable side effects associated with damage to the amygdala. For example, Mark and Ervin have written:

> Tiny electrodes are implanted in the brain and used to destroy a very small number of cells in a precisely determined area. As a surgical technique, it has three great advantages over lobectomy: it requires much less of an opening in the surfaces of the brain than lobectomy does; it destroys less than one-tenth as much brain tissue; and once the electrodes have been inserted in the brain, they can be left without harm to the patient until the surgeon is sure which brain cells are firing abnormally and causing the symptoms of seizures and violence. (Mark and Ervin, 1970, p. 70)

Elsewhere, I have critically examined the biological approaches to the problem of violence in a much more comprehensive way than is possible here (Valenstein, 1973). In this symposium I chose to limit myself to an evaluation of brain stimulation as a means of determining the cause of violent behavior in those individuals displaying a high incidence of such behavior. It will be recalled by the participants at the symposium that there was considerable discussion on this point. Dr. Ervin maintained that he and Dr. Mark did not mean to imply that electrical stimulation can be used in this way, while I maintained that if this is true their book certainly gave the wrong impression to most readers. For example, after describing the initiation of rage and violence by amygdala stimulation in a patient, Mark and Ervin state: "To our knowledge, this is the first time that rage behavior was artificially produced by electrical stimulation in an abnormal brain and used to diagnose the proper placement for a therapeutic lesion" (Mark and Ervin, 1970, p. 108). The implication of such statements is clearly reflected in the consent form used by Ernst Rodin in the much-publicized "John Doe" case at the Lafayette Clinic in Detroit:

> Since conventional treatment efforts over a period of several years have not enabled me to control my outbursts of rage and anti-social behavior, I submit an application to be a subject in a research project which may offer me a form of effective therapy. This therapy is based upon the idea that episodes of anti-social rage and sexuality might be triggered by a disturbance in certain portions of my brain. I understand that in order to be certain that a significant brain disturbance exists, which might relate to my anti-social behavior, an initial operation will have to be performed. This procedure consists of placing fine wires into my brain, which will record the electrical activity from those structures which play a part in anger and sexuality. These electrical waves can then be studied to determine the presence of an abnormality.
>
> In addition, electrical stimulation with weak currents passed through these wires will be done in order to find out if one or several points in the brain can trigger my episodes of violence or unlawful sexuality. In other words this stimulation may cause me to want to commit an aggressive or sexual act, but every effort will be made to have a sufficient number of people present to control me. If the brain disturbance is limited to a small area, I understand that the investigators will destroy this part of my brain with an electrical current. If the abnormality comes from a larger part of my brain, I agree that it should be surgically removed, if the doctors determine that it can be done so, without risk of side effects. Should the electrical activity from the parts of my brain into which the wires have been placed reveal that there is no significant abnormality the wires will simply be withdrawn.
>
> I realize that any operation on the brain carries a number of risks which may be slight, but could be potentially serious. These risks include infection, bleeding, temporary or permanent weakness or paralysis of one or more of my legs or arms, difficulties with speech and thinking, as well as the ability to feel, touch, pain and temperature. Under extraordinary circumstances, it is also possible that I might not survive the operation.
>
> Fully aware of the risks detailed in the paragraphs above, I authorize the physicians of Lafayette Clinic and Providence Hospital to perform the procedures as outlined above. (*Kaimowitz v. Department of Mental Health*, Civil No. 73-19434-AW, Cir. Ct., Wayne County, Michigan, July 10, 1973)

It would appear that there is sufficient confusion to justify some further discussion.

To begin, it should be recognized that preconceived notions about the brain site most likely to be the cause of violent behavior will clearly influence the placement of electrodes. This is especially true where the EEG does not provide unambiguous data for localizing an abnormal site. Clearly, the whole brain can not be sampled. Typically, Mark and Ervin place two electrode assemblies in the temporal lobes on each side. Although each assembly has a number of stimulating electrode tips along its length, it is evident that the amount of the amygdala, not to mention the rest of the brain, that can be examined is limited. Undoubtedly, the placement of the electrode assemblies has been carefully considered in order to obtain the best general representation of temporal lobe electrical activity; but with respect to any individual patient's presumed brain pathology, the electrodes are not likely to be optimally positioned. This problem is compounded if it is decided to destroy an area of the brain, as this is usually accomplished by using the same electrodes to make radio frequency lesions. The site of the lesion, therefore, is restricted to areas surrounding the path of the electrode assemblies.

To turn to the matter of brain stimulation and evoked violence, it is not clear from the literature what success can be expected even with aggressive patients. Chapman (1958) for example, was clearly disappointed in the ability of electrical stimulation to elicit assaultive behavior:

> Some of the clinical features of temporal lobe epilepsy may be reproduced by electrical stimulation of the amygdaloid nuclear region. This was true in five out of six of our patients. The one major feature of their illness that could not be reproduced was assaultive behavior. In no instance was any subjective or behavioral response evoked that remotely resembled aggressiveness. This finding was disconcerting as the major reason for selecting these patients for the electrical coagulation was intractable assaultiveness.

Although Chapman had difficulty eliciting assaultive behavior by amygdala stimulation even in aggressive patients, Kim and Umbach report very different results. Comparing the effectiveness of amygdala stimulation to evoke aggressive behavior in violent and nonviolent patients, they concluded that "aggressiveness increased, whereas no aggressive reaction was observed in non-violent cases. Thus the amygdaloid complex seems not to be specific for anxiety alone or for aggression alone, and shows no specificity of the subnuclei for these emotional states" (Kim and Umbach, 1973, p. 184). Apparently, stimulation of many different nuclei within the amygdala elicited aggressive reactions, but only in patients inclined toward violence.

Putting aside questions about the incidence of evoking aggression by brain stimulation, there remains the matter of interpretation. It should be obvious that it is not safe to attribute any behavior evoked by brain stimulation to the neural area surrounding the electrode tip. Electrical stimulation activates cells located at great distances from the electrode. The delays normally occurring between electrical stimulation and any behavioral consequences are sufficiently long to make it impossible to rule out transmission to any brain area. Plotnik (1974) has analyzed some of the records presented by Mark and Ervin and noted that the evoked behavior may occur as long as 90 to 150 seconds after the stimulation has ended. Plotnik concludes that "the elicited behavior does not, by any stretch of the imagination, closely follow the brain stimulation." An example of the temporal relationship between brain stimulation and assaultive behavior can be seen in the following description of a patient's response:

> Following the termination of the stimulus she relatively slowly over many seconds exhibited the progressively increasing electrical and clinical abnormalities with loss of response to the examiner as noted on the tracings, culminating in a directed attack against the wall, which she suddenly pounded furiously with her fists. This coincided with a maximal burst of high voltage spike-like deflections in the right amygdala and hippocampus. The final excerpt of the sequence shows the reversion of the record toward the pre-stimulation pattern 5 mins. later at which time she was talking coherently. A similar kind of attack with the same electrical features was provoked by such stimulation of the most anterior electrode in the amygdala on the following day. This time she suddenly swung her guitar past the nose of her astonished psychiatrist, smashing the expensive instrument against the wall. On each of the 2 occasions the electrical buildup of abnormality followed the same crescendo pattern, about 2 mins. elapsing in both instances before the maximal electrical, typical seizure outburst coinciding with the furious attack. (Sweet, Ervin, and Mark, 1969, p. 340)

Also to be noted in the above quotation is the fact that more than one electrode elicited the same behavioral response. It will be recalled that Kim and Umbach (1973) observed similar results. The importance of this point becomes clearer from the experimental brain stimulation studies on animals. A few years ago, my colleagues and I placed several stimulating electrodes in different areas of the hypothalamus of rats and reported an interesting trend (Cox and Valenstein, 1969). It was observed that in a number of animals the same response was evoked from very different brain areas, while in other animals either different, or no specific behavior, was elicited from electrodes that appeared to be in comparable brain areas. We concluded that within certain anatomical limits, a "prepotent response" tendency of the animal appeared to be a more important determinant of the behavior evoked than the exact location of the electrode in the brain (Valenstein, 1969).

Subsequently, additional information has accumulated supporting our conclusion. In a recent study, it was noted that in some monkeys, drinking was elicited by a number of electrodes located at very different brain sites. Stimulation at similar sites in other monkeys did not produce any drinking. Apparently, some monkeys respond to brain stimulation at many different sites by drinking, while others do not show this tendency at all (Bowden, Galkin, Rosvold, in press). A similar conclusion may be drawn from an earlier study by Wise (1971), in which rats were implanted with electrodes capable of being moved within the brain after implantation. It was found that in some rats, as the electrode was advanced over a large dorsoventral extent of the hypothalamus, eating and drinking were continuously evoked, but in other rats, these behaviors were not observed in response to stimulation at any site.

Panksepp (1971) has provided other data supporting the "prepotency hypothesis." After studying the elicitation of mouse-killing responses in rats, he concluded that the ability to elicit this behavior by brain stimulation "interacted with the behavioral typology of individual animals, animals normally inclined to kill mice were more likely to kill during hypothalamic stimulation than nonkillers. Thus, the electrically elicited response was probably not determined by specific functions of the tissue under the electrode but by the personality of the rat" (Panksepp, 1971, p. 327).

These experimental results supporting the "prepotency hypothesis" certainly do not mean that stimulation at any brain site will always evoke the same behavior in a particular animal. There can be no questioning the fact that there is much evidence that two or more electrodes can evoke different behaviors from a single animal. The relevant point is that many electrodes evoke states that are not very specific, and therefore an animal's behavioral tendencies (and also the environmental conditions) can be major determinants of the effects produced by stimulation. In many instances, such factors may be more revealing than the exact placement of the electrode tip.

One of the factors that surely must determine whether aggressive behavior is elicited by electrical stimulation is the motivational state that is evoked. Plotnik (1974) has summarized the motivational consequences of 174 brain stimulation sites in monkeys. The motivational effects were determined by tests that measured whether an animal sought out, escaped from, or was indifferent to the brain stimulation. It was found that 117 sites were neutral, 22 were positive or rewarding, and 35 were aversive or negative. All of the 14 points that elicited aggressive behavior directed at other monkeys had aversive motivational properties. Plotnik views the elicited aggression as "secondary aggression" produced by reaction to an aversive stimulus. In such cases, it would be misleading to conclude that there was a direct relation between natural aggression and the brain site stimulated as there would be to conclude the same about the soles of the feet because an electric shock delivered to them produces fighting between animals caged together. The point is well illustrated by Black and Vanderwolf's (1969) report that "foot thumping" could be evoked in the rabbit by stimulation of very diverse brain sites (in the hypothalamus, thalamus, central grey, septum, reticular formation and fornix-fimbria). Rather than postulating the existence of a complex "thumping circuit" in the rabbit brain, the investigators noted that thumping could be elicited by foot shock and they concluded that "thumping behavior in the rabbit is a fear or pain response."

Two factors clearly emerge even from this cursory review of the experimental brain stimulation literature. One of these is that the response tendencies of the subject is a major determinant of the behavior that is evoked by stimulation. The other point is that the emotional state initiated by the stimulation will influence which of the response tendencies of the subject will be expressed. There is little justification for the belief that brain stimulation is a valid technique for locating discrete foci that trigger violence even when such foci exist. In the assaultive patients that are referred to Mark and Ervin, it is likely that violence can be triggered from a great number of brain sites and probably also by a pinch on the skin. There are clearly good reasons for questioning the ability of stimulation techniques to ferret out a "critical focus."

The same conclusion might have been reached by a careful reading of the case histories of the patients involved. It could be seen from this evidence that only bilateral lesions produced any lasting effect (Mark, Sweet and Ervin, 1972). At the very least, it is clear that no single focus was found.

The above conclusion receives additional support from the observation that lesions are made progressively larger until the desired behavior change is believed to have been achieved. It is difficult to be certain about the amount of tissue destroyed because the published records have not presented an adequate amount of detail. The operations in which favorable results are claimed all involve bilateral destruction of temporal lobe tissue. Commonly, a series of destructive lesions are made, but no estimate of the average amount of total tissue destruction has been provided. The information is described in a very general manner: "These lesions were usually made in and around the amygdala in a sequential manner. After the first set of lesions, the electrodes were usually left in place for 1 month or up to one year while we determined if more lesions were needed" (Mark, Sweet and Ervin, 1972, p. 144). Little additional information is available even in the individual case descriptions that are published. The point is especially important because there has been an implicit assumption that the small amount of tissue destroyed in these operations would not have significant consequences for the emotional and intellectual capacities of the patients. We are told that the surgery does not improve any behavioral abnormalities (other than assaultive behavior) that were present preoperatively: "we are commenting mainly about their [the operations'] effect on the episodes of uncontrolled fear, rage, or assaultive behavior. We discerned no effect on other manifestations of psychosis or behavioral abnormalities that may have been present preoperatively" (Mark, Sweet and Ervin, 1972, p. 147). However, insufficient postoperative information has been provided to be certain that no significant personality or intellectual impairment has followed the operation. There are a few scattered comments that seem to suggest some emotional changes produced by the operation. For example, one patient experienced an agitated depression "requiring electroshock and drug treatment for its alleviation," which was not described as part of the preoperative syndrome. It is evident to anyone reading this literature critically that the published information does not provide an adequate basis for conclusions about the postoperative adjustment of the patients.[1]

Although electrical recording information is used to supplement stimulation data, it should not be presumed to eliminate the problems that have been discussed. Moreover, recording from depth electrodes also has its limitations. Ajmone Marsan and Abraham (1966), for example, have observed that abnormal electrical discharge may not be evident in the recording from a depth electrode located only one centimeter away from a focus. There seems to be agreement that ictal, rather than inter-ictal, electrical activity provides the more reliable information, but even during a clinical seizure clear-cut localization signs may be absent (Ajmone Marsan, personal communication, October 10, 1974). Since the violent behavior seen in Mark and Ervin's patients is said to occur between seizures, it is necessary to question the diagnostic value of the electrical recording information obtained.

Not the least of the problems is the existence of multiple foci and the difficulty in determining which of these, if any, may be causally related to the violent behavior. This difficulty is illustrated in a patient described by Mark, Sweet and Ervin (1972). In this fifty-four-year-old epileptic woman a site in the Ammon's horn that "showed a disturbing amount of spiking" was not destroyed because of the fear of further worsening an already significant memory loss (she previously had a unilateral anterior temporal lobectomy). In spite of this, the woman was said to have had the greatest decrement in assaultive behavior of the patients reported in that series.

It appears, therefore, that the use of brain stimulation, and perhaps also depth-recording techniques, to localize discrete foci causing behavior problems has serious limitations. Conclusions about localization drawn from brain stimulation, particularly, can be very misleading if it is assumed that sites capable of evoking pathological behavior are normally the cause of that behavior. A less obvious conclusion is that in spite of all the sophisticated telestimulation and recording techniques employed, the surgery performed does not seem to have differed significantly either in reported success or in amount of tissue destroyed from the amygdalectomies performed by those who do not utilize chronic electrodes (see Valenstein, 1973, for a review).

Lastly, although we may be frustrated by the inability to introduce appropriate social changes to decrease violent behavior, there is certainly no reason to believe that biological solutions will soon be available. While there will continue to be a few assaultive patients with clear brain pathology who may be significantly improved by surgical intervention, for the foreseeable future we should increase, rather than decrease, attempts to find social solutions for what are primarily social problems.

NOTE

[1] Dr. Ernst Rodin (Professor of Neurology, Wayne State University), a co-author of a proposed experiment to compare the effectiveness of amygdalectomy and anti-androgens on incarcerated individuals, reported at a symposium of the Michigan Neuroscience Society (Ann Arbor, Michigan, May 12, 1973) that he was misled by Mark and Ervin's *Violence and the Brain*. Rodin visited Dr. Mark's project in Boston "to obtain the most up-to-date information on the results of surgery for aggressive behavior in human beings," but was disturbed by the disparities between the published accounts and the information available at first hand. (See also Memorandum from Dr. Ernst Rodin to Dr. J.S. Gottlieb, August 9, 1972, submitted as Exhibit AC-4 in *Kaimowitz v. Department of Mental Health*, Civil No. 73-19434-AW [Cir. Ct., Wayne County, Michigan, July 10, 1973].)

REFERENCES

Ajmone Marsan, C., and Abraham, K. Considerations on the use of chronically implanted electrodes in seizure disorders. *Confin. Neurol.*, 1966, *27*, 95-110.

Black, S.L., and Vanderwolf, C.H. Thumping behavior in the rabbit. *Physiol. Behav.*, 1969, *4*, 445-449.

Bowden, D.M., Galkin, T., and Rosvold, H.E. Plasticity of the drinking system as defined by electrical stimulation of the brain (ESB) in monkeys. *Physiol. Behav.*, in press.

Chapman, W.P. Studies of the periamygdaloid area in relation to human behavior. In H.C. Solomon, S. Cobb, and W. Penfield (eds.), *The Brain and Human Behavior. Res. Publ. Assoc. Nerv. Ment. Dis.*, Vol. 36. Baltimore: Williams & Wilkins, 1958, pp. 258-270.

Cox, V.C., and Valenstein, E.S. Distribution of hypothalamic sites yielding stimulus-bound behavior. *Brain Behav. Evol.*, 1969, *2*, 359-376.

Crichton, M. *The Terminal Man*. New York: Alfred A. Knopf, 1972.

Eibl-Eibesfeldt, I. Aggression in the !Ko-Bushman. In S.H. Frazier (ed.), *Aggression, Res. Publ. Assoc. Res. Nerv. Ment. Dis.*, Vol. 52. Baltimore: Williams & Wilkins, 1974, pp. 1-18.

Gloor, P. Discussion. In C.D. Clemente and D.B. Lindsley (eds.), *Aggression and Defense, Neural Mechanisms and Social Patterns*. Los Angeles: University of California Press, 1967, pp. 116-124.

Goldstein, M. Brain research and violent behavior. *Arch. Neurol.*, 1974, *30*, 1-35.

Kim, Y.K., and Umbach, W. Combined stereotaxic lesions for treatment of behavior disorders and severe pain. In L.V. Laitinen and K.E. Livingston (eds.), *Surgical Approaches in Psychiatry*. Baltimore: University Park Press, 1973, pp. 182-188.

Mark, V.H. Psychosurgery versus anti-psychiatry. *Boston Law Review*, 1974, *54*, 217-230.

Mark, V.H., and Ervin, F.R. *Violence and the Brain*. New York: Harper & Row, 1970.

Mark, V.H., and Sweet, W.H. The role of limbic brain dysfunction in aggression. In S.H. Frazier (ed.), *Aggression, Res. Publ. Ass. Res. Nerv. Ment. Dis.*, Vol. 52. Baltimore: Williams & Wilkins, 1974, pp. 186-198.

Mark, V.H., Sweet, W.H., and Ervin, F.R. The effect of amygdalectomy on violent behavior in patients with temporal lobe epilepsy. In E. Hitchcock, L. Laitinen, and K. Vaernet (eds.), *Psychosurgery*. Springfield, Ill.: Charles C. Thomas, 1972, pp. 139-155.

Panksepp, J. Aggression elicited by electrical stimulation of the hypothalamus in albino rats. *Physiol. Behav.*, 1971, *6*, 321-329.

Plotnik, R. Brain stimulation and aggression: Monkeys, apes, and humans. In R.L. Holloway (ed.), *Primate Aggression, Territoriality and Xenophobia: A Comparative Approach*. New York: Academic Press, 1974, pp. 138-149.

Reeves, A.G., and Plum, F. Hyperphagia, rage and dementia accompanying a ventromedial hypothalamic neoplasm. *Arch. Neurol.*, 1969, *20*, 616-624.

Rodin, E.A. Psychomotor epilepsy and aggressive behavior. *Arch. Gen. Psychiat.*, 1973, *28*, 210-213.

Sweet, W.H., Ervin, F. and Mark, V.H. The relationship of violent behavior to focal cerebral disease. In S. Garattini and E.B. Sigg (eds.), *Aggressive Behavior*. New York: John Wiley & Sons, 1969, pp. 336-352.

Turnbull, C.M. *The Mountain People*. New York: Simon & Schuster (Touchstone), 1972.

Valenstein, E.S. Behavior elicited by hypothalamic stimulation: A prepotency hypothesis. *Brain Behav. Evol.*, 1969, *2*, 296-316.

Valenstein, E.S. *Brain Control: A Critical Examination of Brain Stimulation and Psychosurgery*. New York: John Wiley & Sons, 1973.

Wise, R.A. Individual differences in effects of hypothalamic stimulation; The role of stimulation locus. *Physiol. Behav.*, 1971, *6*, 569-572.

The 47, XYY Chromosomal Abnormality: A Critical Appraisal with Respect to Antisocial and Violent Behavior

SALEEM A. SHAH
Chief, Center for Studies of Crime and Delinquency
National Institute of Mental Health
Rockville, Maryland

Even though the study of sex chromosome aneuploidies in humans has occupied geneticists since 1959, during the late 1960's certain aspects of human genetics received considerable scientific as well as popular attention. More specifically, a number of researchers reported an association between antisocial and aggressive behavior and the XYY chromosomal constitution. These reports were followed by considerable mass media publicity about a few accused murderers who were reported to have XYY karyotypes (Shah, 1972).

Despite the biased nature of the populations surveyed in most of the earlier studies (i.e., inmates of prisons, mental hospitals, and maximum security hospitals for mentally disordered offenders), and also the conceptual and methodological problems in many of these studies, some investigators concluded that the extra Y chromosome in some manner predisposed such individuals to engage in antisocial and unusually aggressive behavior (see, for example, Casey et al., 1966;

Forssman and Hambert, 1967; Nielsen, 1968; and Price and Whatmore, 1967).

Some writers stated that it was "reasonable to suggest that [the] antisocial behavior [of the XYY males] is due to the extra Y chromosome" (Price and Whatmore, 1967). Another investigator was moved to state, "It seems unlikely that punishment of any kind would change the risk of new crimes in patients [XYY males] who are genetically predisposed to criminality" (Nielsen, 1968). The term "supermale" was used by another researcher in referring to persons with the 47,XYY complement (Telfer, 1968). Moreover, on the basis of the phenotypic characteristics of tallness, long extremities, facial acne, mild mental retardation, a history of mental illness and criminal behavior, this investigator concluded that Richard Speck—the convicted murderer of eight Chicago nurses—was likely to have an XYY constitution. Indeed, based on some newspaper reports, several writers in the scientific as well as popular press described Speck as an XYY male. Richard Speck seemed to have had the dubious distinction of being cited as though he were the prototypical XYY male. However, later newspaper reports[2] indicated that Speck did *not* have an XYY karyotype. More recently the cytogeneticist who conducted chromosomal studies reported that Speck had a normal 46,XY complement (Engel, 1972).

One might well ponder the irony of the situation in which the individual repeatedly cited as having the *typical* XYY phenotype turned out *not* to have this karyotype at all! Of course, many other writers were urging caution with regard to premature and possibly erroneous conclusions on the basis of preliminary findings obtained from special and selected populations (e.g., Kessler and Moos, 1970; Shah, 1970). It would appear, however, that the professional and career contingencies which influence the publishing behavior of scientists seem often to facilitate a rush to publish novel and dramatic findings.

The tendency to seek premature closure on the issue of the XYY phenotype and various behavioral manifestations seems still not to have abated. Despite the conceptual and methodological problems inherent in most of the studies involving special institutionalized populations, references still appear emphasizing the "unusually aggressive temperament" and the "excessive episodic aggressiveness" of many XYY males (e.g., Jarvik et al., 1973; see also Shah and Borgaonkar, 1974). Yet the available evidence does *not* justify such a description of XYY males. Such a conclusion is especially unwarranted if XYY males are compared with XY controls from the same

[2] For example, Chicago *Herald Tribune*, November 26, 1968.

subpopulations. This does not in any way deny, however, that rather serious medical, psychiatric, behavioral and social pathologies have been noted in many persons with XYY karyotypes. Rather, the point is simply that males with this chromosomal constitution cannot as an entire group be described on the basis of characteristics that may be displayed by only some members of the group.

This discussion will focus on a critical evaluation of the available evidence with respect to assertions about the association of the XYY complement with antisocial, unusually aggressive and violent behavior. Following a brief report on the prevalence estimates for this anomaly, the major findings relevant to socially deviant and violent behaviors will be discussed. Readers interested in a more comprehensive discussion of the general topic of the XYY chromosomal constitution may wish to study several recent reviews (e.g., Baker, 1972; Borgaonkar and Shah, 1974; Hook, 1973; and Owens, 1972).

PREVALENCE ESTIMATES

Several earlier reports have used a prevalence rate of one 47,XYY case in about 700 males (see, for example, Baker, 1972; Hook, 1973; Jacobs et al., 1971). However, on the basis of more recent estimates Borgaonkar and Shah (1974) have suggested that the frequency of the XYY anomaly in the general population would appear to be in the range of one such case in 1,500 to 3,000 males.

Using the latter prevalence rates for the general population unselected for height (i.e., not restricted to only tall males), it is evident that many of the studies of special populations in penal, mental and maximum-security institutions have found higher prevalence rates. Since tallness appears to be a phenotypic trait that appears fairly consistently to be associated with the XYY complement, prevalence rates must be distinguished in terms of whether or not the population surveyed was selected for tallness. For example, Baker (1972) reported a prevalence rate of .125% for "normal adults" screened *without* any selection for height, and a rate of .304% for tall males.

As indicated, several studies of special populations have reported prevalence rates higher than those estimated for the general male population. However, given the very low base rates for the XYY condition, very large numbers of cases must be screened in order to establish significant differences. Thus while the prevalence rates for this condition obtained in mental hospitals and penal institutions have fairly consistently been higher, they have typically not been significantly so. It must be noted, however, that several studies have found remarkably higher prevalence rates (from *two to more than twenty times higher*) among residents of maximum security mental hospitals (see, for example, Jacobs et al., 1971). These are facilities which typically house individuals who have displayed both antisocial (criminal) behavior as well as psychiatric disturbance.

Such findings, along with the elevated prevalence rates among several of the studies on penal populations, have led some authors to assert an association between the XYY condition and antisocial, criminal and/or violent behavior. However, even brief reflection will indicate the logical and conceptual problems in attempting to establish such direct associations.

One does not have to be a criminologist to know that a very small fraction of all criminal behavior comes to official attention. Of the law-violating acts that do come to attention, only a small proportion lead to criminal convictions. Moreover, of all those who are convicted of criminal acts only a small proportion are given prison terms; an even smaller and highly selected group ends up in special security hospitals during some stage of the criminal justice or civil legal processes. Obviously, therefore, inmates of prisons, mental hospitals, and especially of security mental hospitals constitute a very small and highly biased sample of all those who have engaged in and also been officially apprehended for criminal behavior. And since intellectual, social and economic factors are known to be highly related to the probabilities of making an exit from or proceeding further into the criminal justice process, it is obvious that persons who tend to have intellectual, educational, social, economic and other disadvantages are at a greater risk for coming to official attention, as well as for receiving criminal convictions and penal sentences. Therefore, one *cannot* generalize from the findings on inmates of penal or special security hospitals to the very large group of individuals who come to official attention for their criminal acts—let alone to all those who engage in criminal acts but manage to escape detection. (For further discussion of this point see Shah, 1972; Borgaonkar and Shah, 1974.)

BEHAVIORAL CHARACTERISTICS[3]

There are many difficulties in attempting to study genetic factors in various physical characteristics such as height, endocrine, cardiac, neurological and other features. Nevertheless, these problems tend to pale in comparison with the immense complexities involved in seeking

[3] For a more detailed review and discussion of the material that follows see Borgaonkar and Shah, 1974.

to develop adequate genetic hypotheses in regard to behavior. With few exceptions, there are no genes as such for behavior. Genes operate at the molecular level of organization, and the pathways from genes to behavior are mediated through the successively complex intermediaries of enzymes, hormones and neurons (Fuller and Thompson, 1960). Several basic characteristics of human behavior need to be kept in mind with respect to the discussion that follows.

Most behavioral traits of social importance are typically manifested along a continuum. Rarely can natural dividing lines be readily established between the "normal" and "abnormal" range of the particular behavioral spectrum. When such distinctions are drawn for various purposes they will tend generally to be arbitrary and to be based on a variety of social criteria and considerations. These criteria will be located somewhere on a continuous gradation along such axes as "aggressive-nonaggressive," "violent-nonviolent," and "sexually deviant-sexually normal."

Another characteristic of human behavior is its remarkable *fluidity* and its *malleability* by external circumstances. Moreover, a particular sample of behavior needs to be viewed and understood in reference to its particular social and environmental context. Behavior is neither fixed nor absolute, and seldom does it involve only the individual. Rather, behavior should be viewed as involving an interaction between an individual and a particular environment. To varying degrees, the physical and social environment influences the kind of behavior that is displayed. Thus behavioral manifestations such as aggression, altruism, friendliness, irritability, and so forth are not unvarying characteristics of an individual, but are differentially evoked and stimulated by varying types of social, situational and other environmental factors. Clearly, individuals also differ in their propensities for engaging in these and other behaviors.

Another outstanding characteristic of human behavior is its *complexity*. There are rarely any natural or readily apparent basic units of behavior. Behavioral traits can be fragmented along many dimensions and at several levels of analysis—e.g., biochemical, biophysical, psychological, and topographic. In addition, the intricacies of gene-to-behavior pathways make the distinctions between genotype and phenotype especially crucial to formulations in the area of behavioral genetics (see, for example, Fuller, 1957; Thompson, 1957; Gottesman, 1968). There is the additional fact that phenocopies of multi-determined traits such as aggression, impulsivity and deviant sexual response are readily to be found—especially among groups such as convicted and incarcerated offenders.

It will, therefore, usually be very difficult to be sure whether a given phenotypic feature attributed to germinal mutation is neither a phenocopy nor the result of somatic mutations, or is not due to complex recombination phenomena. Moreover, to take a particular (and perhaps relatively infrequent) sample of an individual's *behavior* as it occurs in a particular situational context, to label the behavior as "aggressive," and then to take the further step of labeling the *individual* as "generally aggressive," must be viewed as a beguilingly simple approach and one which does injustice to the complex and dynamic nature of human behavior.

The foregoing discussion bears on the fact that a particular genotype will typically result in a wide range of phenotypic manifestations. A single genotype that largely determines the way in which the organism responds to a particular environment might be associated with an infinite number of environments (Fuller and Thompson, 1960). Stated differently, the genotype determines the norm of reaction or a reaction range.

Gottesman (1966) has suggested that in order to conceptualize the contribution of heredity to a trait such as intelligence, one may think of heredity as fixing a *reaction range*. Within this framework, a genotype may be viewed as determining an indefinite but nevertheless circumscribed assortment of phenotypes. Each phenotype may be viewed as corresponding to one of the many environmental regimes to which the genotype could be exposed. The concept of reaction range should be kept in mind during the following discussion of some of the behavioral characteristics reported to be associated with the 47,XYY chromosomal constitution.

PERSONALITY

Since the earliest reports on males with an XYY karyotype there have been various descriptions of the outstanding personality and behavioral characteristics of such individuals. Since the bulk of the studies have involved rather selected groups (e.g., incarcerated offenders, patients in maximum security hospitals, etc.), a rather wide range of personality and psychiatric problems have been noted.

Hope, Phillips and Loughran (1967) studied the psychological characteristics of the XYY patients discovered at the State Hospital at Carstairs by Jacobs et al. (1965) and further investigated by Price et al. (1966). Seven of the XYY patients were compared with eleven controls from the same institution, who were matched with respect to date of admission to the hospital and legal classification. A variety of psychological tests were administered to both groups to assess personality characteristics such as hostility, direction of hostility, dependence, overreactivity and other traits. Overall, there were very few significant differences between the mean test scores obtained by the two groups. Of the forty-four variables that were examined, only five showed significant differences. The XYY males were viewed as being somewhat lower in self-esteem and more obsessive or introverted. These patients also described themselves on the tests as slower and more cautious in making decisions. There were no marked differences in intelligence, hostility, nor in regard to the direction of expression of hostility—i.e., whether hostile feelings were expressed inwards against the self or outwards against other persons.

The most extensive and adequately controlled psychological study of XYY males to date appears to be that done by Little (1968). Seventeen XYY patients at the maximum security hospital at Rampton were compared with an equal number of non-XYY patients at the same institution. The control group was matched with the index cases on the variables of age (within two years), length of stay at the hospital (plus or minus six months), and I.Q. (plus or minus five points on the verbal scales of the Wechsler Adult Intelligence Scale). In addition to studying a wide range of background and social materials, four psychological tests were also used: 1) Eysenck Personality Inventory; 2) Cattell's 16 Personality-Factors; 3) Rosenzweig's Picture-Frustration test; and 4) the Edwards Personal Preference Schedule (EPPS).

Of the forty-six variables examined, only two showed significant differences between the mean scores of the two groups. On the EPPS the XYY males were significantly higher (at the .05 level) on *Endurance*—i.e., the control subjects tended to describe themselves as having less persistence at jobs of work or problems, and as being easily distracted. On the Cattell 16 P-F test there was a significant difference on *Scale O*, which assesses the bipolar trait of "Confident-Adequacy vs. Guilt Proneness." Essentially, the control subjects tended to score themselves as worrying and anxious, easily upset, hypochondriacal, lonely and brooding. While there were some differences in the psychological tests used by the investigators, in terms of the personality traits being assessed and the direction and nature of the differences obtained, Little's findings are generally consistent with those of Hope, Phillips and Loughran (1967).

On the basis of the studies that have been reported thus far, it would seem that when XYY males have been compared with controls from the same subpopulation, there do *not* appear to be any major differences in personality characteristics as measured by various psychological tests. Indeed, the few significant differences that have been noted certainly do *not* fit the stereotype of the XYY individuals as highly impulsive, aggressive and disturbed, as compared with XY controls from the same population.

PSYCHIATRIC HISTORY AND CHARACTERISTICS

Since the highest prevalence rates for the XYY complement have so far been found in security hospitals and related facilities housing mentally disordered offenders, there has understandably been much discussion of the psychiatric disorders in persons with this chromosomal constitution. The major findings to be discussed here will focus mainly on the relatively larger studies (rather than those describing just two or three cases), and also studies that have attempted to compare the XYY males with controls from the same population.

The nature and range of psychiatric disturbances reported for XYY patients appear to cover a variety of disorders. However, given the very nature of the subpopulations studied, it is hardly surprising that the XYY males located in mental hospitals, penal and special security institutions have been found to display a variety of antisocial and psychiatric symptoms—any more than one would be surprised at findings of depressed intelligence and various organic pathologies among residents of institutions for the mentally retarded.

Much interest, and even more speculation, was stimulated by the report by Price and Whatmore (1967) that among nine XYY males studied at the Carstairs Security Hospital, in only one case were they able to find a severely disturbed family background. In contrast, a much greater proportion of the eighteen randomly selected controls had familial incidence of criminal offenses. Presumably on the basis of this and other findings Price and Whatmore were led to conclude: "There is no reason to believe that these patients (the XYY males) would have indulged in crime had it not been for their abnormal personalities. There is no predisposing family environment, and their criminal activities often start at an age before they are seriously influenced by factors outside the homes" (p. 536).

Aside from the highly questionable assumptions and inferential processes displayed by this statement, it should suffice to note that the above findings regarding a so-called lack of familial criminological background have not been corroborated by several other investigators (see, for example, Clark et al., 1970; Little, 1968; Nielsen, 1970). For example, Little (1968) found no significant differences with respect to the incidence of crimes in the families of seventeen XYY males and the matched non-XYY controls from the same institution. In addition, this investigator was unable to find any marked difference in the quality and stability of family background between the two groups.

Price and Whatmore (1967) also reported that all nine of their XYY patients at Carstairs had a severe degree of personality disorder, and that they showed extreme instability and irresponsibility. However, the meaning and validity of this statement has to be tempered by the fact that the great bulk of the patients in this security hospital (i.e., 74%) had been classified as suffering from "Severe Personality Disorder," and thus presumably were about equally disturbed. It is noteworthy that six of the nine index patients had histories of court commitments to institutions for the mentally subnormal, as compared with only three of the 18 controls.

Griffiths et al. (1970) found statistically significant differences (.02 level) with respect to the extent of previous psychiatric history in comparing nine XYY prisoners and matched controls. There was a greater incidence of a past history of mental illness among the index cases, and such illnesses were often severe and usually designated as psychopathy. In addition, the XYY prisoners tended to have more frequent histories of attending schools for maladjusted children, as well as histories of truancy and school expulsion. Furthermore, the XYY males had a greater frequency of "serious accidents" (1.3 versus 0.4) as compared to the controls.

Casey (1969) reports that the proportion of families with a mentally ill or mentally subnormal parent or sibling was very similar among the XYY, XXY, and random control patients. "Mental illness" was defined as admission to a mental hospital or inpatient psychiatric facility. Mental subnormality was similarly defined in terms of admission to a special school or occupation center, or registration as a mental defective.

Another rather interesting finding reported by Casey (1969) was that in regard to mental illness, mental subnormality, and criminality in other family members, a sibling was more commonly affected than a parent. The presence of such behavior problems among the siblings would appear to suggest some familial predisposition rather than chromosomal abnormality. Casey also found that over half the families in the three groups (XYY, XXY and control patients) had a family history of either disturbed behavior, mental disorder or parental loss. If the chromosomal abnormality was a major variable predisposing to such disturbed behavior, a lower incidence of disturbed family background might have been expected.

Finally, Little's study (1968) also revealed few differences among the XYY patients and matched and random controls on behavioral as well as background data. The XYY criminals were not different from the

XY criminals on various familial, background, and offense histories, and personality characteristics. It would appear, then, that there were relatively few differences between the XYY and the XY "psychopathic" offenders studied by this investigator. However, many more such studies are needed, and studies involving larger numbers of cases in a variety of subpopulations, before reliable and meaningful conclusions can be drawn. However, the range and inconsistency of the findings that have already been obtained does point to the fact that it is difficult at this point to assert very many definite conclusions about the personality and psychiatric characteristics of XYY males. It seems evident that when mentally disturbed XYY patients have been compared to matched controls *from the same population*, there appear to be very few significant differences.

It would appear that the earlier findings and conclusions regarding severe personality disorders by Price and Whatmore (1967) are not supported by several other studies. Moreover, this writer must confess his perplexity in trying to understand how exactly Price and Whatmore were led to their rather bald conclusion: "All the data we have obtained from the examination of the XYY males at the State Hospital at Carstairs led us to believe that the extra Y chromosome has resulted in a severely disordered personality, and that this disorder has led these men into conflict with the law" (p. 536).

Since these investigators had noted earlier in their paper that fully 74% of the population at Carstairs had been diagnosed as suffering from "severe personality disorders," and since the vast majority of such individuals did *not* have gonosomal aneuploidies, it is difficult to understand the inferential logic that enabled these authors to conclude that "the extra Y chromosome [has] resulted" in the personality disorder.

SOCIAL AND CRIMINOLOGICAL FINDINGS

This section will address the available evidence with respect to antisocial and criminal behavior, viz., in reference to speculations and assertions about the greater aggressiveness and violence of XYY males. The major focus will be on seven larger reports relevant to this issue (viz., Casey, 1969; Griffiths et al., 1969 and 1970; Hope, Phillips and Loughran, 1967; Little, 1968; McKerracher, 1971; Price and Whatmore, 1967; and Street and Watson, 1969).

Criminal History and Types of Crimes

Price and Whatmore (1967) compared the criminal behavior of nine XYY males with eighteen controls (seventeen of these having XY karyotypes) in the same institution. The penal records of the XYY males included considerably *fewer* crimes of violence against persons, but were of comparable length. Griffiths et al. (1969) compared nine XYY prisoners with an equal number of matched XY prisoners and found significant differences (.02 level) with respect to the mean number of previous convictions (13 versus 9.2). Age at first conviction and number of offenses did not show differences, nor did total length of previous penal sentence.

Street and Watson (1969) found some interesting but not statistically significant differences in the patterns of previous offenses committed by XYY, XXY and XY patients in a security hospital. Patients with sex chromosome aneuploidies were most often involved in sexual offenses—59% of the XYY subjects, 56% of the Klinefelter cases, and 34% of the XY controls. There were no discernible differences with regard to nonsexual offenses against persons and property offenses. Interestingly, when offensive behavior immediately prior to admission to the security hospital (Rampton) was considered (excluding behaviors that had not resulted in prosecution), the XY controls were found to have been involved in more nonsexual aggression towards persons (58%) than XYY patients (32%), and the XXY patients (37%). This difference was statistically significant (.05 level).

In comparing incarcerated prisoners with XYY and XXY karyotypes Clark et al. (1970) were not able to find any discernible differences in the records of criminal convictions nor in the types of crimes committed. In contrast, Nielsen (1970) did find differences among XYY (N=12) and Klinefelter males (N=61) from psychiatric and medical wards, a forensic psychiatric ward, an institution for criminal psychopaths, and a sample of "unselected" Danish men. The XYY males in this rather mixed group of cases had a greater frequency of violent crimes (36%), as compared to the XXY males (4%), and the general proportion of sentences given for violent crimes in Denmark in 1966 (13%). Also, the frequency of sexual crimes (including such crimes against children) was distinctly higher among the Klinefelter males (43%) and the XYY subjects (45%) than in mentally retarded male patients (25%), males with borderline intelligence (35%), and a group described as "unselected Danish men" (14%). It must be noted with respect to this particular report that, given the rather motley collection of samples combining the cases from these different groups, it is difficult to know just what significance can be attached to these findings.

An interesting comparison was made by Casey (1969) of the chromosomally abnormal and control patients at Rampton who also had histories of criminal convictions among other family members. The purpose was to see if there were any striking differences in the criminal behavior of the chromosomally abnormal and control patients and the offensive behavior of their family members. There was an increased proportion of sexual offenses in the Rampton patients in comparison to their families: 37.5% of the XYY patients (three of eight) were involved in sexual offenses as compared to only 12.5% of their families. Similarly, 40% of the control patients (six of fifteen) had been involved in sexual offenses as compared to 20% of their families. In contrast, fully 70% (seven of ten) Klinefelter patients had been involved in sexual crimes as compared with only 10% of their families.

In contrast to the above findings, Little (1968) did not find any differences in regard to the specific offenses committed by 17 XYY, 17 matched non-XYY, and 34 randomly selected patients at Rampton. McKerracher (1971) studied the same patient groups but classified the various offenses into eight broad (and somewhat overlapping) categories—namely, sex offenses of any kind, aggressive sex, interpersonal aggression, aggression of any kind, larceny, breaking and entering, absconding, and a miscellaneous category. The rationale for using this classification was to subsume the offense behavior under general patterns of reaction, such as aggressive, sexual and acquisitive. When the above classification was used two significant differences emerged. Both groups of patients with sex chromosome aneuploidies had a greater proportion of convictions for sexual crimes (60% of both XYY and XXY patients), as compared with 39% of the XY controls. The index patients had a lower proportion of assaultive offenses (excluding sexual aggression): 35% of the XYY cases, 42% of the Klinefelter patients, as compared with 63% of the controls.

The above findings must be interpreted with caution. It is clear that the results that have been discussed tend to vary from study to study, but that some consistent differences in the pattern of offenses are suggested. However, the differences appear to fluctuate depending upon the particular group of patients studied, and also depending on the manner in which the categories of criminal behavior are classified. Since in many instances the eventual criminal charges may not reflect accurately the actual offense behavior (because of the lack of reliable or legally sufficient evidence, the precise nature of proof required to obtain convictions for particular offenses, and also possible changes in criminal charges as a result of "plea bargaining"), some degree of variation is certainly to be expected. Despite all these caveats, it is noteworthy that the available evidence certainly does *not* support assertions that XYY males as a group are more likely to engage in unusually aggressive and violent crimes as compared with XY males from the same study populations.

Institutional Behavior and Adjustment

There are many uncertainties concerning the antisocial behaviors that actually occur in the free community. Much of the criminal behavior goes unreported; some of the reported behavior may fail to have proper substantiation and legally sufficient evidence; it is also very difficult to determine the social and environmental context in which the behavior occurred—for example, whether a criminal assault and battery was unprovoked, was instrumental to obtaining a victim's money, or whether it was in response to some provocation or even in self-defense. Hence, information about the institutional behavior and adjustment of patients in closed institutions helps to provide somewhat more meaningful and reliable information. Such behavior is more readily detected, the social and situational factors are easier to elucidate, and the comparisons among different groups are somewhat more meaningful—since all the behaviors take place within the same restricted and closed environment.

It may be recalled that Price and Whatmore (1967) reported that the *control patients* in the Carstairs study were more openly hostile and displayed more violently aggressive outbursts in the hospital than did the XYY patients.

Street and Watson (1969) investigated the institutional adjustment of XYY (N=22), XYY (N=16), and XY control (N=50) patients at Rampton; an abundance of evidence was obtained to support and further add to the brief reference to hospital adjustment made by Price and Whatmore. Street and Watson found rather interesting and also statistically significant differences on a number of behavioral indices. The XYY and XXY patients tended to form better relationships with the staff than did the controls. Specifically, 90% of the XXY patients, 81% of the Klinefelter males, and only 54% of the controls were rated as forming "good relationships with staff." In contrast to several other reports (e.g., Daly, 1969), very few of the patients with sex chromosome abnormalities (9% of the XYY and none of the Klinefelter males) formed homosexual liaisons with other patients in the hospital, as compared with 38% of the control patients. This was a statistically significant difference.

There were also a number of other rather interesting findings. The *control* patients were involved in more aggression against staff (26%) as compared with 9% of the XYY and 11% of the XXY patients. Similarly, the *control* patients displayed more aggression against other patients (56%) as compared with the XYY (37%) and XXY (28%) patients. In view of the popular speculation about the so-called greater aggression and violence of XYY males, and also since these patients were significantly taller (mean height 71.33 inches) as compared to the XXY males (mean height 68.25 inches), and the control patients (mean height 67.37 inches), somewhat more—not less—aggressive behavior towards others might possibly have been expected.

Other findings reported by Street and Watson (1969) point to the better adjustment and less disruption by the XYY patients in the hospital. Greater instability was displayed by the control patients at Rampton, as judged by their higher rate of failure in the Villa Wards (presumably the less secure and more privileged sections of the hospital) and return to the Block Wards. Such returns to the Block Wards occurred in 14% of the controls but in only 7% of the XYY males. Furthermore, better behavior and adjustment in the hospital by the XYY patients is indicated by the fact that they showed less need for psychotropic medication (only 15% of the group) as compared to the control patients (32%).

Finally, and possibly reflecting the better relationship with the staff and other patients and their overall adjustment, the XYY (as well as the XXY) patients had a shorter average length of stay at the hospital (6.7 and 6.9 years, respectively), as compared to the control patients (average stay of 8.2 years). There was no appreciable difference in the readmission rates to the hospital for the XYY, XXY, and control patients (18%, 22%, and 20%, respectively).

Overall, then, the available data indicate the generally better institutional behavior and adjustment shown by the XYY (and XXY) patients in security hospitals when compared to the adjustment and behavior of the XY controls in the same facilities.

The findings that have been analyzed in the preceding discussion do *not* provide support for the conclusion that XYY males involved in trouble with the law are any more aggressive, violent, and impulsive as compared with XY controls from the same population.

In order to check the assertion that XYY males were predisposed in some fashion to engage in antisocial and violent behavior, Clark et al. (1970) compared a number of XYY and XXY males in penal institutions. Little difference was found between the pattern of behaviors displayed and past criminal records. These authors were led to conclude: "While a more extensive and thorough study of this new minority group is needed, it now appears that in general the XYY male has been falsely stigmatized. The frequency of his involvement in antisocial behavior and crime may not be appreciably different from that of the average citizen" (p. 1662).

In light of the findings that have been discussed in the preceding section, an additional point might be added to the conclusion stated by Clark et al. The frequency of antisocial and violent behavior by XYY males is probably not very different from that of non-XYY males of similar background and social class and located in the same subpopulations (that is to say, prisons, mental hospitals, and security institutions).

CONCLUSION

No simple relationship can be established between certain classes of socially deviant behavior and the official handling and designations of the individuals as criminals or mental patients. Variables pertaining to socioeconomic status are deeply embedded in the societal processes for the definition and handling of deviant behaviors. The more skilled and resourceful law violators have a lower probability of being apprehended, and even when apprehended, they have lower probabilities of being convicted and sentenced to penal or other institutions. In the subpopulation of incarcerated offenders, persons from the lower social classes and those who have relatively greater biologic, psychologic, social and economic handicaps will tend typically to be overrepresented. Moreover, such socially disadvantaged groups tend to have higher frequencies of pre- and postnatal health, nutritional, and related problems, as well as higher incidences of pregnancy and birth complications, and what Montagu (1972) has referred to as a "social deprivation syndrome." (For more details on this point see Shah and Roth, 1974.)

It might also be recalled that Robinson and Puck (1965 and 1967) have reported that sex chromosome aneuploidies may occur with greater frequency in families with a depressed socioeconomic status. Similarly, problems associated with a general "social deprivation syndrome" will also tend to occur with increased frequency in such families.

There are, therefore, many conceptual, logical, as well as empirical problems in attempting to attach simple and direct causal relationships between the presence of an extra Y chromosome and confinement in certain public institutions. This is not said to deny in any way the importance of genetic variables in affecting human behavior. Rather, it is simply being emphasized that the complexities of genotypic and environmental interactions, and the as yet undetermined ways in which the influence of the extra Y chromosome may be mediated, do *not* allow simplistic causal assertions.

It would be misleading and even erroneous to consider the genetic contributions of relevance to the XYY phenotype as being unvarying or absolute. Phenotypic characteristics are determined as a result of interactions between the genotype and its environment. In the earlier reference to Gottesman's concept of *reaction range*, it was mentioned that each phenotype corresponds to one of several possible environmental regimes to which the genotype could be exposed. Given exposure to a very different environment, the same genotype could be expected to develop differently. Thus, to demonstrate that there is a genetic contribution to psychopathy, for example, warrants only the hypothesis that in certain environments, some genotypes respond by developing a variety of behavioral problems more frequently than other genotypes. This hypothesis does not preclude the possibility that in some other environments the same genotype may yield individuals with better regulated and more socially adapted behaviors.

Given the abundance of evidence pointing to the phenotypic heterogeneity associated with the 47,XYY chromosomal constitution, it becomes essential to consider the mediating effects of numerous other variables. Assuming some "vulnerability" transmitted via the extra Y chromosome, one still has to consider the various interactions of the genotype with the intrauterine and postnatal environments, e.g., the exogenous influences of infections, radioactivity, malnutrition, other toxic effects, and perinatal complications. In addition, there are the numerous postnatal interactions of the developing organism with its physical and social environment. Even assuming a definite "vulnerability" associated with the XYY constitution, such a potential may become overtly manifested, and even seriously exacerbated, in environments in which family instability, inadequate parental supervision, and other forms of social stress abound. The same "vulnerability" might fairly adequately be compensated for in more positive and supportive familial and social environments.

For example, there have been numerous reports relating a disturbed family background to an increased incidence of behavior problems among youngsters with epilepsy and various EEG abnormalities (e.g., Grunberg and Pond, 1957; Ounsted, 1969; Taylor, 1969; and Weiss et al., 1971). In fact, Stevens, Sachdev and Milstein (1968) found that adverse family environment led all other predisposing factors in differentiating behavior problem children from controls—even though almost half (47%) of the index children had distinctly abnormal EEG tracings. Similarly, there have been several reports that individuals with sex chromosome aneuploidies who have been in trouble with the law often came from disturbed family backgrounds (e.g., Casey, 1969; Clark et al., 1970; Nielsen, 1970).

In view of the phenotypic heterogeneity that is clearly associated with the 47,XYY chromosomal constitution, it would be erroneous to suppose a definite and narrow range of phenotypic variation; or to assume the existence of a particular XYY syndrome. More importantly, since certain types of scientific findings and conclusions have rather important implications for social policy decisions, it certainly behooves researchers to exercise proper caution in interpreting data from preliminary studies and selected population samples with respect to the XYY anomaly. Regretably, such scientific caution has not been evidenced in many instances in regard to assertions concerning the behavioral characteristics of persons with an XYY chromosomal constitution.

REFERENCES

Baker, D. Chromosome errors and antisocial behavior. *CRC Critical Reviews in Clinical Laboratory Sciences*, January 1972, 41-101.

Borgaonkar, D.S., and Shah, S.A. The XYY chromosome male—or syndrome? In A.A. Steinberg and A.G. Bearn (eds.) *Progress in Medical Genetics*. Vol. 10. New York: Grune & Stratton, 1974, pp. 135-222.

Casey, M.D. The family and behavioral history of patients with chromosome abnormality in the special hospitals of Rampton and Moss Side. In D.J. West (ed.) *Criminological Implications of Chromosome Abnormalities*. Institute of Criminology, University of Cambridge, 1969, pp. 40-60.

Casey, M.D., Segall, L.J., Street, D.R.K., and Blank, C.E. Sex chromosome abnormalities in two state hospitals for patients requiring special security. *Nature*, 1966, 209, 641-642.

Clark, G.R., Telfer, M.A., Baker, D., and Rosen, M. Sex chromosomes, crime, and psychosis. *American Journal of Psychiatry*, 1970, *126*, 1659-1663.

Daly, R.F. Mental illness and patterns of behavior in 10 XYY males. *Journal of Nervous and Mental Diseases*, 1969, *149*, 318-327.

Engel, E. Guest editorial: The making of an XYY. *American Journal of Mental Deficiency*, 1972, *77*, 123-127.

Forrsman, H., and Hambert, G. Chromosomes and antisocial behaviour. *Excerpta Criminologica*, 1967, *7*, 5ff.

Fuller, J.L. The genetic base: pathways between genes and behavioral characteristics. In *The Nature and Transmission of the Genetic and Cultural Characteristics of Human Populations*. New York: Milbank Foundation, 1957, pp. 101-111.

Fuller, J.L., and Thompson, W.R. *Behavior Genetics*. New York: Wiley, 1960.

Gottesman, I.I. Genetic variance in adaptive personality traits. *Journal of Child Psychology*, 1966, *7*, 199-208.

Gottesman, I.I. A sampler of human behavioral genetics. In T. Dobzhansky, M.K. Hecht, and W.C. Steere (eds.), *Evolutionary Biology*, 1968, *2*, 276-320.

Griffiths, A.W. Prisoners of XYY constitution; psychological aspects. *British Journal of Psychiatry*, 1971, *119*, 193-194.

Griffiths, A.W., Richards, B.W., Zaremba, J., Abramowicz, T., and Stewart, A. An investigation of a group of XYY prisoners. In D.J. West (ed.), *Criminological Implications of Chromosome Abnormalities*. Institute of Criminology, University of Cambridge, 1969, pp. 32-43.

Griffiths, A.W., Richards, B.W., Zaremba, J., Abramowicz, T., and Stewart, A. Psychological and sociological investigation of XYY prisoners. *Nature*, 1970, *227*, 290-292.

Grunberg, F., and Pond, D.A. Conduct disorders in epileptic children. *Journal of Neurology, Neurosurgery and Psychiatry*, 1957, *20*, 65-68.

Hook, E.B. Behavioral implications of the human XYY genotype. *Science*, 1973, *179*, 139-150.

Hope, K., Phillips, A.E., and Loughran, J.M. Psychological characteristics associated with XYY sex chromosome complement in a state mental hospital. *British Journal of Psychiatry*, 1967, *113*, 495-498.

Jacobs, P.A., Brunton, M., Melville, M.M., Brittain, R.P., and McClemont, W.F. Aggressive behavior, mental subnormality, and the XYY male. *Nature*, 1965, *208*, 1351-1352.

Jacobs, P.A., Price, W.H., Richmond, S., and Ratcliff, R.A.W. Chromosome surveys in penal institutions and approved schools. *Journal of Medical Genetics*, 1971, *8*, 49-58.

Jarvik, L.F., Klodin, V., and Matsuyama, S.S. Human aggression and the extra Y chromosome: fact or fantasy? *American Psychologist*, 1973, *28*, 674-682.

Kessler, S., and Moos, R.H. The XYY karyotype and criminality: a review. *Journal of Psychiatric Research*, 1970, *7*, 153-170.

Little, A.J. Psychological characteristics and patterns of crime among males with an XYY sex chromosome complement in a maximum security hospital. Unpublished dissertation for the B.A.Sp. Hons. degree, Sheffield University, 1968.

McKerracher, D.W. Psychological aspects of a sex chromatin abnormality. *Canadian Psychologist*, 1971, *12*, 270-281.

Montagu, A. Sociogenics. *American Anthropologist*, 1972, *74*, 1025-1061.

Nielsen, J. The XYY syndrome in a mental hospital: genetically determined criminality. *British Journal of Criminology*, 1968, *8*, 186-202.

Nielsen, J. Criminality among patients with Klinefelter's syndrome and the XYY syndrome. *British Journal of Psychiatry*, 1970, *117*, 365-369.

Ounsted, C. Aggression and epilepsy: rage in children with temporal lobe epilepsy. *Journal of Psychosomatic Research*, 1969, *13*, 237-242.

Owens, D.R. The 47,XYY male: a review. *Psychological Bulletin*, 1972, *78*, 209-233.

Price, W.H., Strong, J.A., Whatmore, P.B., and McClemont, W.F. Criminal patients with XYY sex-chromosome complement. *Lancet*, 1966, *i*, 565-566.

Price, W.H., and Whatmore, P.B. Criminal behaviour and the XYY male. *Nature*, 1967, *213*, 815.

Robinson, A., and Puck, T.T. Sex chromatin in newborns: presumptive evidence for external factors in human nondisjunction. *Science*, 1965, *148*, 83-85.

Robinson, A., and Puck, T.T. Studies on chromosomal nondisjuction in man. II. *American Journal of Human Genetics*, 1967, *19*, 112-129.

Shah, S.A. *Report on the XYY Chromosomal Abnormality*. Public Health Service Publication No. 2103. Washington, D.C.: U.S. Government Printing Office, 1970.

Shah, S.A. Recent developments in human genetics and their implications for problems of social deviance. *Birth Defects Original Article Series*, 1972, 8, 42-82.

Shah, S.A., and Borgaonkar, D.S. The XYY chromosomal abnormality: some "facts" and some "fantasies"? *American Psychologist*, 1974, *29*, 357-359.

Shah, S.A., and Roth, L.H. Biological and psychophysiological factors in criminality. In D. Glaser (ed.), *Handbook of Criminology*. Chicago: Rand McNally, 1974, pp. 101-173.

Stevens, J.R., Sachdev, K., and Milstein, V. Behavior disorders of childhood and the electroencephalogram. *Archives of Neurology*, 1968, *18*, 160-167.

Street, D.R.K., and Watson, R.A. Patients with chromosome abnormalities in Rampton Hospital. In D.J. West (ed.) *Criminological Implications of Chromosome Abnormalities*. Institute of Criminology, University of Cambridge, 1969, pp. 61-67.

Taylor, D.C. Aggression and epilepsy. *Journal of Psychosomatic Research*, 1969, *13*, 229-236.

Telfer, M.A. Are some criminals born that way? *Think*, 1968, *34*, 24-28.

Thompson, W.R. Traits, factors, and genes. *Eugenic Quarterly*, 1957, *4*, 8-16.

Weiss, G., Minde, K., Werry, J.S., Douglas, V., and Nemeth, E. Studies on the hyperactive child. VIII. Five-year followup. *Archives of General Psychiatry*, 1971, *24*, 409-414.

Research Strategies for the Study of Human Violence

ROBERT PLUTCHIK
Albert Einstein College of Medicine
Bronx, New York
CARLOS CLIMENT
Universidad del Valle
Cali, Colombia
FRANK ERVIN
University of California
Los Angeles, California[1]

This paper will present preliminary data obtained through two programs dealing with factors related to violent behavior in individuals. One of these programs focused on violent individuals, self-referred or identified through clinics or physicians. These individuals were to be carefully screened, using extensive medical, neurological, and psychometric indices. The aim was to try to determine what proportion of this violent group, if any, suffered from identifiable brain dysfunction. The second program was established to study patients who had probable or identified brain dysfunction and who also showed episodic outbursts of violent behavior. These patients were to be intensively evaluated in a specially designed hospital ward. The purpose of the present paper is to describe the development of the research methodology, the tests used, and the populations studied, as well as some of the theoretical issues involved, and to report on some of the findings obtained during the first year of the programs.

[1] We should like to thank Mr. James Hovey for assistance in gathering some of the data reported here.

HOW PREVALENT IS VIOLENCE?

A large number of people in America suffer from some form of brain dysfunction. To the two million who have epilepsy must be added the six million mentally retarded, the estimated two and a half million persons with minimal brain disorders, and the unknown number suffering from strokes, tumors, and the like. In addition, many of the estimated two to three million persons who have sustained head injuries through war or automobile accidents have probably developed some degree of brain dysfunction. Recent work has also indicated that protein malnutrition in the infant has long-lasting effects on the developing brain of a child (Coursin, 1968; Mark and Ervin, 1970).

There are many well-documented clinical cases that demonstrate that brain injury or brain disease can create episodic outbursts of anger. Rare cases of tumor and virus infection—e.g., rabies—are dramatic examples of violent behavior resulting from disordered brain function. There is also an extensive animal literature showing that electrical stimulation of certain brain areas will generally produce appropriate attack or destructive behavior (Wasman and Flynn, 1962; Roberts and Kiess, 1964; Delgado, 1966). A connection between altered brain function and violent behavior therefore certainly exists, but a number of important questions are unanswered.

These questions can be explained best by reference to Table 1. It is obvious that a certain proportion of people with brain dysfunction show violent behavior. It is also evident that many people who have no brain disease show violent behavior. There are no currently available data that would enable us to complete this fourfold table. Most probably there will never be a completely satisfactory set of figures for this table. There are two general reasons for this statement: (1) The term "brain dysfunction" is not uniquely definable. It includes such things as gross injuries to the brain, subtle biochemical abnormalities, and microscopic changes in cells. We do not believe prevalence data on such abnormalities will ever be available. (2) The term "violence" is also ambiguous. It is used to describe such diverse events as destructive behavior, angry feelings, fantasies, accidental injuries and indirect attacks on objects. Political radicals have one view of violence, and conservatives another. However, in this study, attention was limited to individuals who exhibited recurrent episodes of attack behavior directed at other individuals.

For every definition of the term that could be created there would

TABLE 1

A basic requirement for a theory of brain-behavior interrelationships is to determine the data needed to complete this table.

DYSFUNCTION	VIOLENCE: YES	VIOLENCE: NO
YES		
NO		

be a different set of numbers in Table 1. Since the term "violence" has so many political implications quite separate from its value as a scientific term, we believe that no universally accepted definition will ever be created.

This conclusion does not mean that the subject of violence and aggression cannot be studied. Quite the contrary. It is worth emphasizing, however, that science does not start with definitions; it ends with them. Science advances only by successive approximations to that ultimately unreachable asymptote called truth.

We do not believe it will ever be possible for anyone to determine causal connections between brain dysfunction and violence in the general population. However, we believe that for specific subgroups of the population we can establish plausible correlations between violent behavior and brain dysfunctions.

This would require using pragmatically relevant definitions of the key terms "violent" and "nonviolent." In time, the number of groups compared will increase, and our measures will also increase in sophistication. If under these conditions we find replication of results when "violent" and "nonviolent" individuals are compared, then our interpretations become increasingly general.

HYPOTHESES OF THE PRESENT STUDY

The present study hoped to identify a group of individuals who are considered by themselves or by their community as violent persons. It was expected on the basis of previous research that these violent individuals would show more medical and neurological abnormalities than any appropriate comparison groups. In general, it was expected that the greater the frequency and intensity of violent behavior shown by a group of individuals, the greater the probability of various other classes of abnormalities, such as medical problems, soft and hard neurological signs, and a history of family psychiatric difficulties (Climent, Rollins, Ervin, and Plutchik, 1973).

In our initial planning of the study we hoped to be able to identify violent individuals through several sources: hospitals, courts, prisons, social agencies and letters to physicians. Extensive diagnostic evaluations of these individuals would be made and the results compared with those obtained from nonviolent individuals. Referrals to our Research Diagnostic Clinic could be from any part of the country. Criteria for acceptance to the clinic would be that violent behavior is present and has proven to be a problem to the patient, his family, or his community. For the initial screening, no formal definition of violence would be used. If the patient or the referring source believed that a problem of violence existed, the clinic would do a diagnostic evaluation.

THE PROBLEM OF CONTROL GROUPS

We spent a good deal of time discussing the question of what would be an appropriate control group for the violent individuals. Should it be a group of ordinary citizens recruited through an ad in the newspaper? Should it be a group of medical students who volunteer to be tested? Will a group of patients in an outpatient clinic make a more appropriate control group? Or should we use the ubiquitous college sophomore? It is obvious that any one of these choices would create possible biases of unknown magnitude, and greatly limit our ability to generalize the findings.

It should also be evident that control groups are points of reference that are relevant to the hypotheses being tested. For example, if the researcher's hypothesis is that a person who attempts suicide is a scapegoat within his own family, then a reasonable control group might be siblings of the suicidal person. However, if the hypothesis is that this suicidal person is temporarily insane, then an appropriate control group might be nonsuicidal admissions to a mental hospital. There is no single control group that would be appropriate for all hypotheses.

This was also the conclusion we came to in our study of violent individuals. We felt that it was, in fact, a fallacy to even talk about control groups in the usual laboratory sense for the following reason. In most clinical studies, we cannot use the laboratory method, which consists of taking a large number of subjects, dividing them randomly in half and administering an experimental condition to one of the subgroups. In clinical research we are forced to use naturally occurring, existing groups as subjects of study. We then make a half-hearted attempt to match the groups on some hopefully relevant variable such as age, race or sex, and then proceed as if the groups are then equal in all important respects.

This method has several important drawbacks: (1) It ignores the fact that matching on a few variables such as age and sex does not equate the groups on dozens of other variables that may in fact be relevant. Matching gives a false sense of security in that differences that are found between the so-called experimental and control groups are mistakenly attributed to the variable of interest (e.g., violence) rather than to many other variables that are not being measured. (2) A second drawback is that matching on some variables sometimes creates marked sampling biases. For example, suppose that violent persons have a lower I.Q. on the average than nonviolent ones. If we attempt to match on I.Q. we will be implicitly selecting the relatively brighter violent subjects and matching them to the relatively duller nonviolent subjects. Neither group will then be particularly representative of its larger population.

Another aspect of the sampling biases created by matching is related to the fact that large numbers of subjects must sometimes be eliminated in the pursuit of matched groups. In one hospital study 500 records were examined in order to find 40 schizophrenics who were matched on age, sex, I.Q., and family income (Kellerman, 1964). The question then arises: if 90 percent of all possible subjects are discarded from the study because they cannot be matched, how representative can the results be? The more variables used for matching, the more unrepresentative are the groups being compared.

Some of these problems have been created by an uncritical transfer of the typical laboratory design to the clinical research context. When we deal with natural groups in clinical settings we can never make causal statements about variables. At best, we can only make plausible statements about possible relations between variables. This aim is by no means trivial, in view of the fact that we can usually think up only a small number of plausible hypotheses to account for a given finding. What is central in clinical research is the nexus of interrelated observations obtained from many groups using multiple measures.

There is one other important point I should like to make concerning the use of multiple comparison groups. It is not enough to compare three or four groups to establish a network of observations. Of even greater importance is the need to establish groups in which there is an implicit scaling of the variable of interest (Plutchik, 1973). To illustrate, if we were interested in suicide, we might compare four groups: (1) a group of persons who make a near-lethal suicide attempt; (2) a group of persons who make a minimally lethal suicide attempt; (3) a group of depressed individuals who make no attempt; and (4) a group of normal individuals. It is not necessary that these groups be matched on age, race, and sex or other variables, except in the rare cases where there is definite evidence that such variables have an effect on the particular measures being used in the study.

In the study of violence which we were planning, we decided to use these ideas as the basis for the selection of groups. We assumed that the self- or medically referred individuals would have the highest scores on our measures of violence. We also assumed that a prison population of men and women would be higher on violence than normal individuals, but lower than our self-referred persons. To obtain a normal group we decided to use a college sample of males and females, but in addition, we decided to try to get each self-referred violent person to bring a friend or acquaintance with him from his own community, who might be willing to take the same tests as the referred patient. (Unfortunately, only one-fourth of the self-referred violent patients brought such a friend and we did not obtain enough data to form a group).

Another group that we believed would represent low overt violence was formerly hospitalized mental patients attending an outpatient clinic. We thus hoped to obtain a number of groups ranging in levels of expressed violence from very high to very low. Each person in each group would be tested on a battery of psychometric instruments, questionnaires, and neurological measures, and averages and correlations would be obtained from this ordered series of groups.

This set of groups that were implicitly scaled on levels of expressed violent behavior would thus hopefully provide a framework for interpreting levels of violence found in other groups less clearly defined on this variable. Therefore, additional information on our battery of psychometric tests was obtained from other groups whose status relative to degree of expressed violence was not known. One of these groups consisted of general neurological patients; another consisted of patients being treated for intractable pain; and the other two groups consisted of temporal lobe or other types of epileptics. The characteristics of the eleven groups studied are given below.

THE COMPARISON GROUPS

(1) *The Self-Referred Violent Persons.* Most of these people came to the Research Diagnostic Clinic because they heard about if from their physicians or social workers; some were referred by emergency room clinics. Over the six-month period that the clinic was actually collecting psychometric data, we were able to interview and test 17 such individuals, 15 men and 2 women. Their mean age was 26 (SD = 7.1).

A case history describing this type of patient is the following. Mr. H.W., at the age of 19, woke one morning in his college dormitory with bruises and a black eye and no memory of any fight. He was evaluated by the college physicians and diagnosed as having temporal lobe epilepsy and placed on medication. His symptoms were thereby controlled and he went on to obtain a master's degree with no further problems.

At the age of 30 he began to have episodes of rage which often resulted in assaults on both his wife and child. He was self-referred to the Research Diagnostic Clinic after an apparent seizure in church followed by assaultive behavior toward his wife and other persons in the congregation.

After screening, H.W. was admitted to the inpatient service where a diagnosis of temporal lobe epilepsy was confirmed. His medication was changed and he was discharged. A follow-up six months later showed no further symptoms.

(2) *The Male Prisoners.* These prisoners were incarcerated at Bridgewater State Hospital Center for Sexually Dangerous Persons. All the men were sentenced there because of sex crimes such as rape or indecent assault on a minor. Permission was obtained from the prison officials to seek volunteers for our interviews and tests. No special privileges were granted to the volunteers, and anonymity was guaranteed. We were able to recruit 23 prisoners, with a mean age of 30 (SD = 5.2), in the six months of testing.

(3) *The Female Prisoners.* These women were incarcerated at the Framingham State Prison for Women. Several studies had been done in the past at this prison and good working relations existed with both the staff and the inmates. We obtained 30 volunteers, with a mean age of 29 (SD = 4.3).

(4) *Boston State Hospital Male Outpatients.* These 13 men were recruited from the outpatient clinic at Boston State Hospital. Almost all had been hospitalized in this state institution previously. Most had the diagnosis of schizophrenia while in the hospital. Their mean age was 38 (SD = 5.8).

(5) *Boston State Hospital Female Outpatients.* These 30 women also were tested at the Boston State Hospital Outpatient Clinic. They too had been mostly diagnosed as schizophrenic while in the hospital. They ranged in age from 26 to 48 with a mean age of 37 (SD = 6.5).

(6) *Male College Students.* There were 83 students who volunteered to take our battery of psychometric tests. These students were in business and sociology classes at Suffolk University in Boston. They completed the forms without any personal identification. The students ranged in age from 18 to 23, with a mean of 20 (SD = 2.8).

(7) *Female College Students.* There were 35 female college students in the Simmons College sample. Their ages ranged from 17 to 23 years, with a mean age of 19 (SD = 2.4).

(8) *General Neurology Patients.* Data on some of the scales in the battery were obtained from 40 general neurology patients at Boston City Hospital. These were patients who were in the clinic for evaluation or treatment of such diverse ailments as disc problems, neuritis, headaches, back pains, etc. They ranged in age from 31 to 63, with a mean of 44 (SD = 6.2).

(9) *Massachusetts General Hospital Pain Patients.* These 17 patients had gone to the Pain Clinic at MGH because of intractable pain due to a variety of medical conditions. The patients ranged in age from 27 to 50, with a mean of 37 (SD = 5.5). Seven of this group were women.

(10) *Boston City Hospital Temporal Lobe Epileptics.* These were patients who had been evaluated at the special epilepsy research clinic at Boston City Hospital. After a diagnostic evaluation, 9 of the patients were believed to possess some form of temporal lobe epilepsy. Six of this group were males. The age range of these 9 patients was 17 to 48, with a mean of 27 years (SD = 7.4).

(11) *Boston City Hospital Non-Temporal Lobe Epileptics.* Of the 21 patients evaluated for epilepsy during the six-month period of testing, 12 patients were diagnosed as having some other form of epilepsy. The mean age of this group was 26 (SD = 3.8). Eight were males.

In summary, in the six months of actual operation of the data-gathering phase of the project, we were able to obtain psychometric information on eleven groups of individuals for a total of 309 people. With the exception of a few black patients in the outpatient groups, all were white. Members of the different groups varied widely in the levels of expressed violent behavior, and also varied in type of brain dysfunction, if any. We expected these eleven groups to provide an interrelated set of comparisons that would help us interpret our findings.

It is worth emphasizing the fact that psychometric data were obtained on 309 people. Our original plan was to use these findings and to relate them to various biomedical indices. Unfortunately, the psychological test data were collected much more rapidly than the medical screening data. Except for a few EEG's and dermatoglyphic measures, the projects were terminated before the medical screening procedures could be instituted. The result is that all the results to be reported here are relations between psychometric variables and group membership, with some tenuous inferences about possible brain-behavior interrelationships.

THE PSYCHOMETRIC VARIABLES

Examination of some of the literature dealing with violent individuals suggested that our problem and approach was almost unique. Most of the literature on human violence is anecdotal, historical, psychoanalytic, or based on social indicators such as crime statistics (Wolfgang, 1958; Mulvihill and Tumin, 1969). Some laboratory studies of aggression describe what college students or children do in mildly frustrating situations. Very little information exists on the natural history of violent individuals as assessed by psychometric instruments.

We expected that the majority of the individuals whom we would wish to evaluate would be of limited educational background; they would probably have difficulty in concentrating, and would probably have low thresholds for boredom and irritability. This meant that the kinds of tests, scales, and questionnaires selected should be relatively brief and structured, and should be directed at variables which previous experience has suggested as fruitful. These brief tests could be interspersed with medical examinations.

We felt no need to rely on psychological tests which had been developed for other populations and purposes, unless they could be shown to relate directly to the variables with which we were concerned. A test such as the MMPI, for example, would not be used in its entirety (over 500 questions) partly because of the length, and partly because most of the scales seemed irrelevant to our needs. No projective tests were to be used because of the excessive amount of time needed for administration, and because of their doubtful relation to the overt behavior in which we were interested. We decided that it would be most fruitful in the long run to construct a number of new scales on which we could collect normative data and which we could validate independently. These were the guidelines which prompted the development and use of a series of tests and scales, all of which could be completed by the patient himself.

Preliminary Clinic Contact Form

This form was to be filled out by the clinic secretary at the time of initial contact. It was designed to provide identification data useful for administrative purposes, as well as some basic medical data.

Personal Background Form

This form consists of fifty questions which have precoded alternative answers available to the patient. The questions concern the medical and family history of the patients. They deal with such content areas as history of psychiatric illness, early signs of violence, personal and family evidence of physical illnesses that have genetic loadings, patterns of driving behavior, criminal behavior, social difficulties, and behavior and symptoms associated with menstruation.

Interview Form

The interview form was developed to obtain information from the patients through the use of a structured interview. The content areas covered in the interview include early childhood experiences, descriptions of parental behavior, frequency of occurrence of family problems regarding school difficulties, violence within the family, marital problems, etc. The final version of the form was put into structured format so that patients could answer the questions without an interviewer present.

FAV Questionnaire

This questionnaire consists of thirty questions concerning feelings and acts of violence. The respondent is asked to indicate whether each description is true for him by using a three-point scale: "Never True," "Sometimes True," or "Often True." An overall score is obtained which reflects an individual's tendency to act violently.

FAS Questionnaire

This questionnaire consists of twenty questions concerning sexual feelings and sexual behaviors. The respondent is asked to indicate whether each description is true for him by using a three-point scale: "Never True," "Sometimes True," or "Often True." An overall score is obtained which reflects the strength of an individual's sexual preoccupation or drive.

Problem Check List

The problem check list is a modified version of the Mooney Check List (Mooney and Gordon, 1950), with an orientation towards more overt psychiatric problems, rather than towards the everyday problems of college students for which the test was originally designed. The test has a series of brief descriptions of problems which people sometimes have—for example, being overweight, being unable to hold onto a job, feeling afraid to speak up, confusion in religious beliefs, losing one's temper too easily, feeling rejected by one's family or embarrassment about sex. The items are actually grouped into seven major content areas: physical symptoms and problems; job problems; personal insecurities; difficulties in interpersonal relations; family problems; religious problems; and sexual problems.

Columbia M-D Scale

This scale was developed as part of a long-term study of manic-depressive patients. It consists of 52 statements about an individual's typical behavior, each of which can be answered as "Yes" or "No." The items can be scored in two categories: those items that discriminate depression from normalcy, and those items that discriminate mania from normalcy. Two scores are thus obtained, a depression score and a mania score (Plutchik et al., 1970).

Monroe Dyscontrol Scale

This scale is based upon the work of neurologist Russell Monroe, whose work concerns episodic behavioral disorders and epilepsy (Monroe, 1970). Monroe reported that a review of his clinical records revealed eighteen statements often made by patients with "epileptoid" impulsive disorders. These statements have been modified and associated with a four-point frequency scale ranging from "Never" to "Often." A single overall score is obtained.

M-M Scales

These scales are a selection of items from the MMPI. The only two MMPI scales that seemed to have special relevance to the objectives of the research project are the Sc or Schizophrenia scale and the Pd or

Psychopathic Deviate scale. However, an examination of the items that comprised these scales indicated that very few had face or content validity for the defined scale, and that the scales were too long (e.g., the Sc scale alone had 78 items). Therefore, 20 items having the highest face validities were selected from each scale and incorporated into this new form. The result is a 55-item test based directly on the MMPI, which provides three scores, a Lie score, a Schizophrenia score, and a Psychopathic Deviate score.

Emotions Profile Index

This index consists of twelve affect words, such as "affectionate," "resentful," and "obedient," which have been paired against each other in all possible combinations to produce 66 pairs. The twelve items have been selected to sample all aspects of the trait or emotion language. Each term has then been coded to represent certain implicit emotional states which have been referred to as primary or prototype emotions in the theory proposed by Plutchik (1962). The theory assumes that all emotions can be conceptualized as mixtures of two or more of eight primary emotions which have certain systematic relations to each other. Since each word on the EPI is scored for these emotion categories, whenever a patient makes a choice of one of the two items in a pair, he is building up a score on the primary emotions. The EPI provides eight emotion scores plus a bias (or social desirability) score (Plutchik, 1970; Plutchik and Kellerman, 1974).

In addition to these self-report scales, two observational instruments were created for use on the hospital research ward.

Seizure Form

This form consists of a series of brief descriptions of behaviors and feelings related to epileptic states. It includes such things as auras, clonic movements, falling, momentary losses of attention, and actual unconsciousness. The form was used to monitor the seizure-related behavior of each patient on the ward. Attendants and nurses were required to determine the applicability of these items to each patient every two and a half hours, or approximately three times during each shift, a total of nine times a day. The judgments represented the pooled information of all staff members on a given shift.

Aggression Form

This form consists of a detailed list of violent behaviors that could be observed on the ward. Each item is descriptive of an overt act and requires a minimum of inference on the part of the observer. Items of the following type are included: hitting someone, breaking windows, threats, attempted rape, suicidal attempts, stealing, refusal to take medication, etc. The items are grouped under a number of major headings: aggression against others, threats, indirect aggression, aggression against self, and social aggression. This form was used to monitor the violent behavior exhibited by each patient on the ward. Attendants and nurses were required to determine the applicability of these items to each patient every two and a half hours, or approximately three times during each shift, a total of nine times a day.

In addition to these two scales, all the other tests used at the Research Diagnostic Clinic were also used on the Research Ward so that comparable data became available.

Finally, a series of brief cognitive paper-and-pencil type tests were developed which we hoped could provide us with some indices of organicity. There were six such tests: Attention-Concentration; Immediate Memory Span; Serial Learning; Interference Sets; Paired Associates; and Paired Symbols. These tests were developed relatively late in the project and were therefore administered to only a few patients. For this reason, no formal statistical comparisons were made.

RESULTS

Group Differences On Selected Variables

The results have been analyzed in two major ways. The first involves a comparison of all groups on each of the 34 variables. Although there are significant differences among the groups on many of these variables, we have selected seven key variables for discussion. These are illustrated in Figures 1 to 7.

Figure 1 shows total scores on the Problem Check List. The temporal lobe epileptics and the violent self-referrals have significantly more life problems (job, family, sex, interpersonal, etc.), than the prisoners and other groups. The college students and general neurology patients have the least number of problems. Although one cannot make causal statements, it is reasonable to hypothesize that there may be some common experiences or common underlying problems in both the epileptic and violent self-referred patients. It is not valid to assume from this figure that the common element is the presence of episodic violence in both groups. This point can be documented in Figure 2.

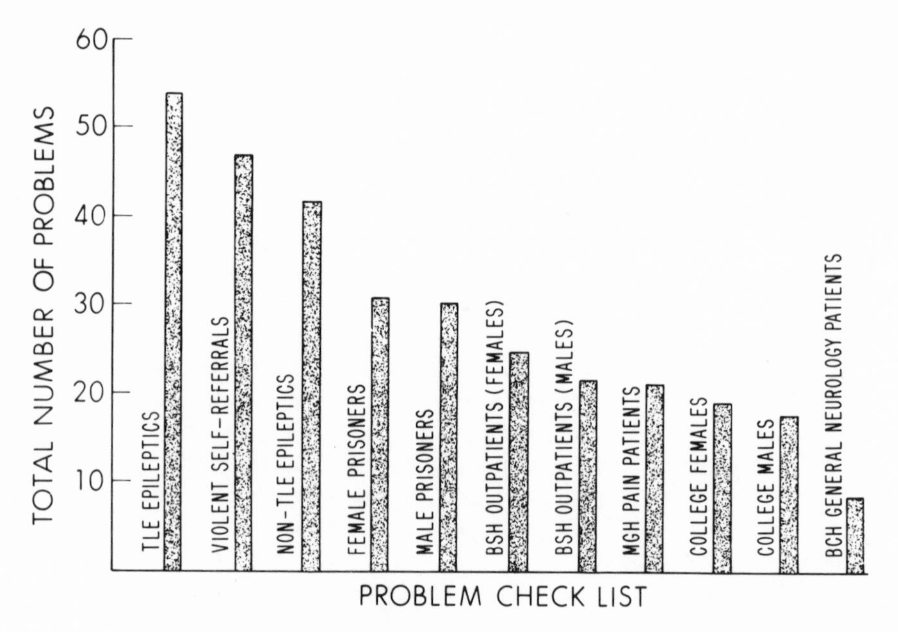

FIG. 1. Mean scores obtained by eleven different groups on total number of problems on the Problem Check List.

The FAV Scale is a direct measure of self-reported violent feelings and acts. The self-referred violent patients score highest on this scale, thus contributing to the face validity of the scale. They are significantly higher than all the other groups except the prisoners. The male and female prisoners also score quite high on the FAV. College males and females fall around the middle of the distribution of groups, and the temporal lobe epileptics fall toward the low end of the scale. The epileptics are thus not violent individuals as assessed by their own self-reports, even though they report a large number of life problems.

Figure 3 shows the distribution of mean scores on the Monroe Dyscontrol Scale. Here again, the face validity of the scale is supported by the fact that the epileptic groups have the highest scores. Close to their scores are those of the violent self-referrals and the male prisoners. The college students and general medical patients are significantly lower than the epileptics. These findings, taken in conjunction with the previous ones, show that the Monroe Scale is measuring something different from violent feelings or behavior. The episodic dyscontrol symptoms which the test purports to measure are apparently highly represented in several diverse groups: epileptics, violent

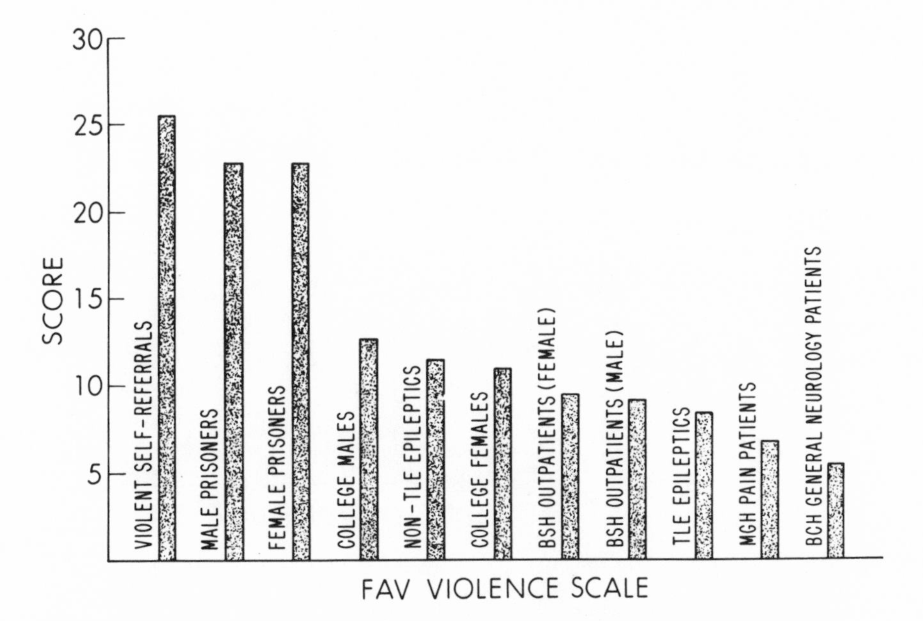

FIG. 2. Mean scores obtained by eleven different groups on FAV self-reported violence scores.

persons and prisoners. Episodic dyscontrol is by no means the same as violent behavior, although the two may often go together.

It has often been stated that sex and aggression are closely interwoven. It was because of this common assumption that we developed the FAS Scale designed to measure feelings and acts related to sex. The FAS can be considered to be a measure of sex drive.

Figure 4 shows that the male prisoners have significantly higher scores on sex drive than any of the other groups. It is interesting to note that the violent self-referrals and the college males have equal FAS scores, and these are noticeably above those of the epileptic groups and the general medical group. It is also worth noting that in each of the three cases where we have a male and female group from the same type of population, the male group is higher on the FAS than the female.

The correlation between mean FAV violence score and mean FAS sex-drive score across the different groups is +.77. This suggests that sex and aggression may be influenced by some of the same factors.

We decided to look at certain personality variables. Figure 5 shows the depression scale percentile scores on the Emotions Profile Index.

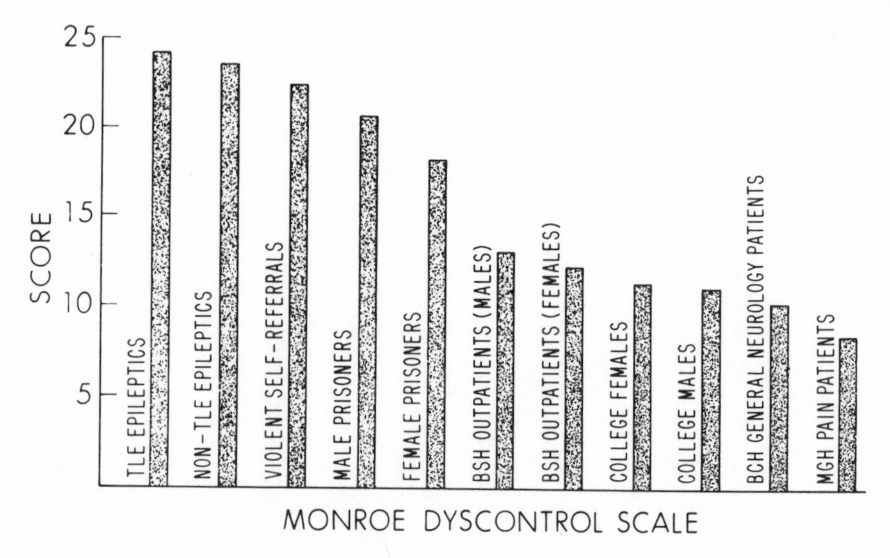

FIG. 3. Mean scores obtained by eleven different groups on the Monroe Dyscontrol Scale, an index of epileptiform symptoms.

The ordering of the groups on depression is quite different for this variable than it is for the others. The female prisoners and the violent self-referrals are most depressed, and the college students are least depressed. The pain patients, the epileptics, and the outpatients tend to fall somewhere in the middle. In a previous study by Climent et al. (1973), female prisoners from the same prison as studied here reported a high percentage of suicidal thoughts and attempts.

Figure 6 shows the scores of each group on the twenty-item Psychopathic Deviate subscale of the MMPI. True to the content validity of the scale, the male and female prisoners obtained the highest mean scores. The male prisoners are significantly higher than any other group. The violent self-referrals are next highest, and the college students and outpatients have the lowest scores. (Unfortunately, we did not obtain information on the temporal lobe patients using this scale). This suggests that the violent self-referred patients tend to act in ways which society defines as psychopathic.

Figure 7 shows the scores of each group on the twenty-item Schizophrenia subscale of the MMPI. The violent self-referred patients score significantly higher than most of the other groups. The Schizophrenia scale contains such items as the following: "Does everything taste the same to you? Do people say insulting and vulgar things about you?"

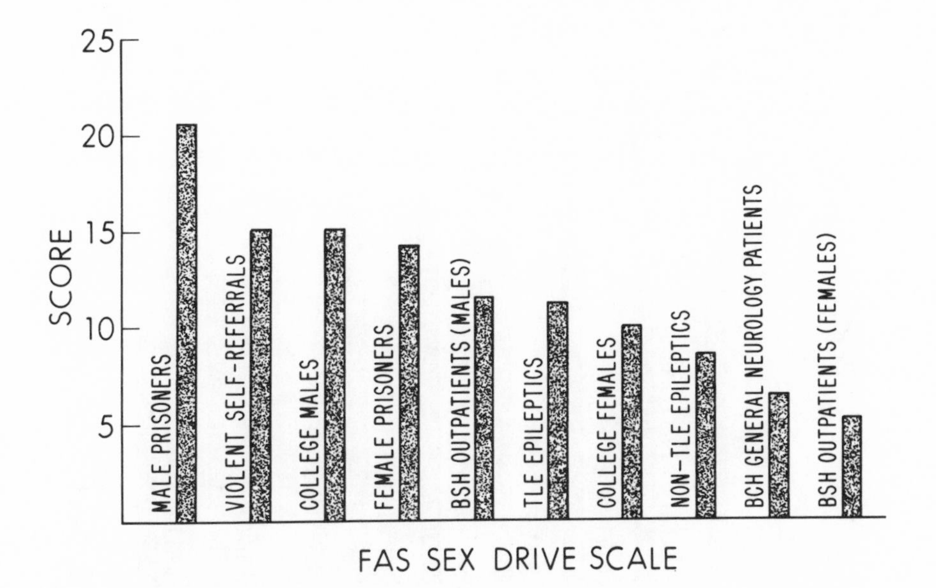

FIG. 4. Mean scores obtained by eleven different groups on the FAS scale, an index of the strength of the sex drive.

"Do you dislike having people near you?" "Do you feel there is something wrong with your mind?" etc. A "yes" answer in each of these cases would contribute to scores on the schizophrenia scale.

The college students show the lowest score, with one exception. The Boston State Hospital male outpatients have the lowest mean score on Schizophrenia. This is surprising in view of the fact that most of the members of this group had been diagnosed as schizophrenics. This apparent discrepancy is made more understandable if we consider the Lie scale of the MMPI. This male outpatient group had the highest score of any group on the Lie scale, thus suggesting maximum defensiveness.

The results obtained with the two MMPI subscales imply that the violent self-referred patients describe themselves in ways that we tend to interpret as both psychopathic and schizoid. It is therefore likely that many such individuals will end up at mental hospitals or in prisons. It will undoubtedly be a difficult diagnostic problem to distinguish "true" schizophrenic individuals from those schizoid persons with dyscontrol problems, although the scale and tests we have described here may be useful in such an undertaking.

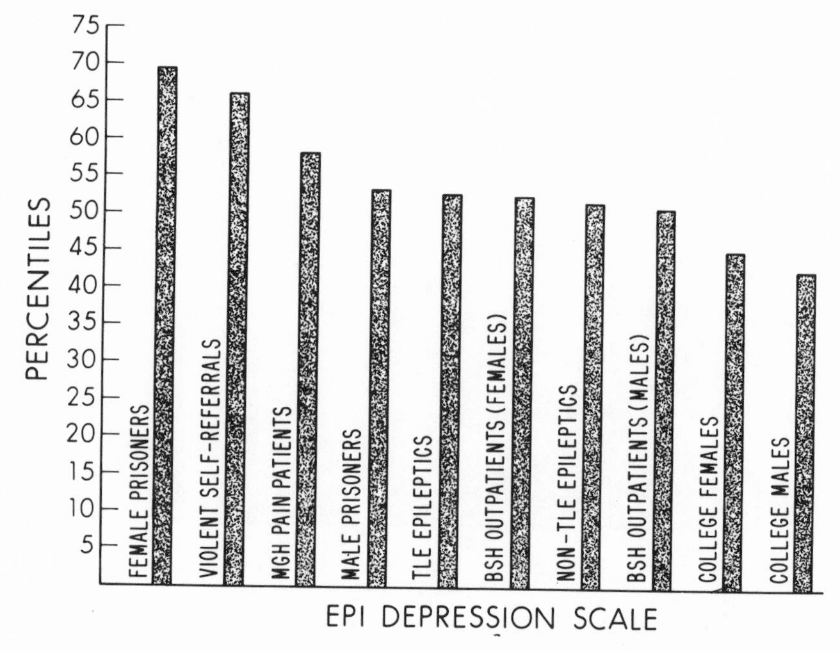

FIG. 5. Mean scores obtained by eleven different groups on the Depression scale of the Emotions Profile Index.

Variables Correlated with Violence or Dyscontrol

The second way in which the data were analyzed was in terms of the variables which are correlated with violence or dyscontrol. For this analysis, intercorrelation matrices were computed for all 34 variables; this was done separately for each of seven groups: the violent self-referred patients, the male and female prisoners, the male and female college students, and the male and female psychiatric outpatients.

All variables which correlated significantly with the FAV violence score and with the Monroe Dyscontrol Scale score were identified. For the sample size of most groups, a correlation of approximately +.40 is significantly different from zero at the 5 percent level.

Examination of the data showed that some of the variables correlated with FAV violence scores in only one group of subjects; however, some variables correlated with FAV scores in two or three or even all seven groups. Since each group is independent of the others, a significant correlation between two variables in two or more groups

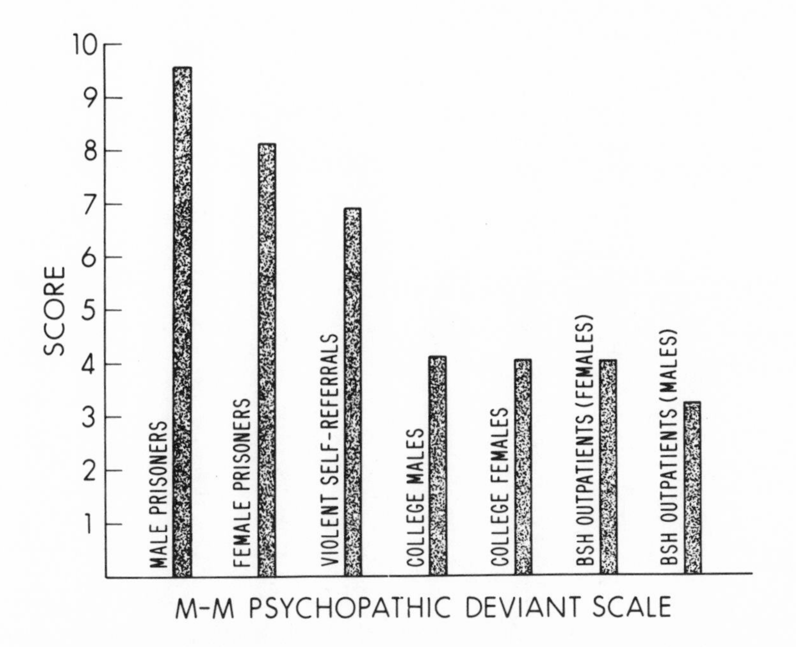

FIG. 6. Mean scores obtained by seven different groups on the Psychopathic Deviate subscale of the MMPI.

represents independent confirmation of a relationship. If the chance probability of finding a certain correlation in each of two independent groups is 5 percent, then the probability of finding the same significant correlation in both groups by chance is the product of the two probabilities, or .0025. The probability of finding a given variable significantly correlated with FAV violence scores *by chance* in seven independent groups, is approximately $(.05)^7$, which makes such a finding extremely unlikely as a chance occurence.

Table 2 presents those variables found to be significantly correlated with FAV violence scores in two or more groups. The mean correlation across the groups, based on Fisher's *z* transformation, is also presented.

The results indicate that a history of family violence correlates with high FAV violence scores in the individual. The term "family violence" is defined by five items of the Personal Background Form, with the following weights assigned: *Never* (0); *Sometimes* (1); or *Often* (2). The five items are

1. When you were a child, were you spanked by your father?

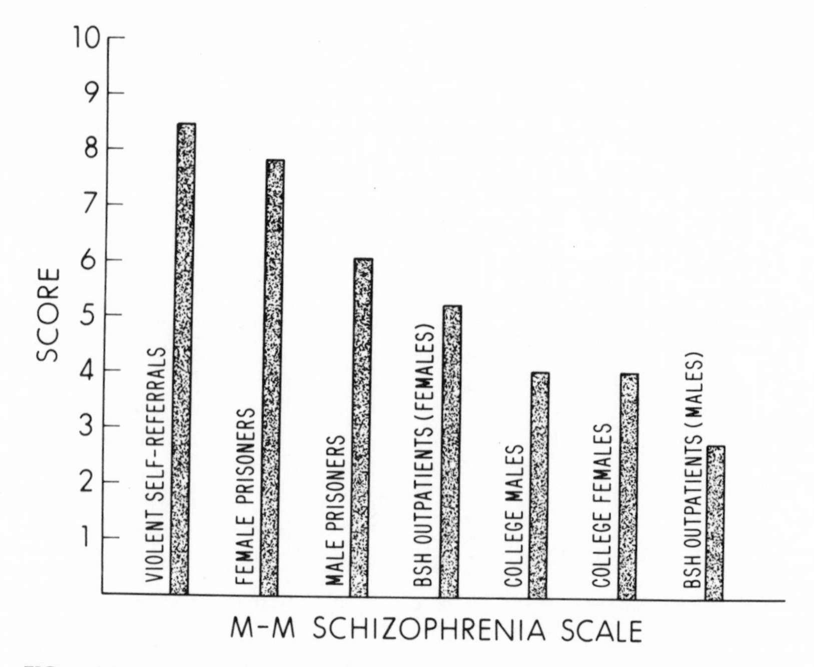

FIG. 7. Mean scores obtained by seven different groups on the Schizophrenia subscale of the MMPI.

2. When you were a child, were you spanked by your mother?
3. When you were a child, did you get into fights with other children?
4. Did you ever observe your parents quarreling?
5. Did you ever observe your father hitting your mother?

Scores on the Monroe Scale also correlated significantly with FAV violence scores in all seven groups. Some positive correlation between these two scales should be expected since six of the eighteen items of the Monroe Scale relate to violent behavior. But most of the items reflect loss of control of oneself (e.g., "I have had sudden changes in my moods"; "I have had blackouts"; "I have been surprised by my actions" etc.).

In five of the seven groups, there is a significant correlation between FAV scores and the total number of problems reported on the Problem Check List. Similarly, in five of the seven groups there is a significant correlation between FAV scores and the total number of behavior problems reported by each individual. (The Problem Check List con-

TABLE 2

Variables Significantly Correlated with the FAV Violence Scale in Two Or More of Seven Groups

Variable	Number of Groups	Mean Correlation
History of Family Violence	7	.42
Monroe Scale (Epileptiform Dyscontrol States)	7	.61
Total Number of Problems (Health, Job, Social, etc.)	5	.39
Number of Behavior Problems (Truancy, Drugs, etc.)	5	.61
Schizophrenia Scale (Subset of MMPI Items	4	.50
FAS Sex Drive Scale	3	.50
Number of Emotional Problems	3	.44
EPI Aggression Score	2	.55
EPI Timidity Score	2	−.39
Number of Behavior Problems In Family Members	2	.53
Psychopathic Deviate Scale (Subset of MMPI Items)	2	.75

sists of 112 items describing possible problems in seven major areas. The Behavior Problem Inventory consists of a list of fifteen serious acting-out behavior problems: learning problem at school; behavior problem at school; truancy, stealing; assaultive behavior; runaway; desertion; hypochondriasis; severe depression; suicidal attempts; hyperactive behavior; temper outbursts; suspicious of other people; drug addiction; and other. The patient is to indicate which of these behaviors he shows, or showed in the past.)

In four of the seven groups, the modified Schizophrenia subscale of the MMPI correlated significantly with the FAV scale, suggesting that people who describe themselves as aggressive on the FAV tend to report other unusual or extreme descriptions of themselves.

Other variables which correlated positively with FAV violence scores are: the FAS sex-drive index; the number of emotional problems on the Problem Check List; the Aggression and Timidity scores (a minus correlation) on the Emotions Profile Index; the number of behavior problems ascribed to family members (based on the fifteen-item list of the Behavior Problem Inventory); and the Psychopathic Deviate subscale of the MMPI. This last-named scale, although correlating with FAV scores in only two groups, has the highest average correlation, namely +.75. Generally speaking, it appears that a large number of life problems in both an individual and his family are the best predictor of a high FAV self-report violence score.

Table 3 lists those variables found to be significantly correlated with the Monroe Dyscontrol Scale. We assume on the basis of the data already presented, that the Monroe Scale is a measure of epileptiform symptoms, and that individuals with high scores on this scale have some likelihood of brain dysfunction. Table 3 shows that the Schizophrenia subscale of the MMPI correlated positively with Monroe Dyscontrol scores in all seven groups. It thus appears that epileptoid dyscontrol symptoms tend to be generally associated with schizoid symptoms. This is consistent with the observation that has often been made that temporal lobe epileptics not infrequently become more schizoid in their behavior as they grow older.

Three variables correlate with Dyscontrol scores in five of the seven groups. These variables are: total number of problems on the Problem Check List; number of problems on the Behavior Problem Inventory; and number of emotional problems on one of the scales of the Problem Check List. Three other sets of problems correlate with Monroe Dyscontrol scores in four out of seven groups. In addition, both a history of family violence and the MMPI subset of items from the Psychopathic Deviate scale correlate with Monroe scores.

Other variables which correlate with Monroe Dyscontrol scores are the FAS sex-drive scale (3 groups); the MMPI Lie scale (3 groups; a minus correlation); the Social Deviance Index; the M-D depression scale; and the total frequency in family members of such diseases as diabetes, migraine headaches, heart disease, cancer, epilepsy, cleft palate, mental retardation, alcoholism, asthma, high blood pressure, ulcers, and drug addiction.

It thus appears that the Monroe Dyscontrol Scale tends to correlate with a group of variables which are fairly similar to those which correlate with FAV violence scores. Generally speaking, the variables correlating with violence include: a family history of violence, a

TABLE 3

Variables Significantly Correlated With The Monroe Dyscontrol Scale In Two Or More Of Seven Groups

Variable	Number of Groups	Mean Correlation
Schizophrenia Scale (Subset of MMPI Items)	7	.42
FAV Violence Scale	7	.61
Total Number of Problems (Health, Job, Social, etc.)	5	.58
Number of Emotional Problems	5	.56
Number of Behavior Problems (Truancy, Drugs, etc.)	5	.53
Number of Health Problems	4	.46
Number of Sexual Problems	4	.62
Number of Social Problems	4	.57
History of Family Violence	4	.56
Psychopathic Deviate Scale (Subset of MMPI Items)	4	.52
Lie Scale (MMPI)	3	−.40
FAS Sex Drive Scale	3	.53
Social Deviance Index	3	.46
M-D Depression Scale	2	.58
History of Family Disease	2	.53

history of many life adjustment problems, a history of acting-out behavior, a tendency toward schizoid thinking, a tendency toward psychopathic behavior, and a tendency toward loss of control.

DISCUSSION

It must be emphasized that the study described here is incomplete. The 309 persons tested represent only a part of those whom we planned to test, and some of the groups are small. Another limitation is that in most cases it was not possible to collect the medical information we desired, for reasons beyond our control. However, because of the nature of the groups and psychometric instruments used, it is possible to present some plausible hypotheses about relations between violence and possible brain dysfunction.

We have found that self-referred (or medically referred) violent individuals have the highest scores on a paper-and-pencil test of violence and also on a test of schizophrenic thinking. They also tend to be quite high on symptoms of epileptic dyscontrol, on frequency of life adjustment problems, on sex drive, on depression, and on psychopathic tendencies.

Those patients who are known to have some form of epilepsy get the highest scores on the Monroe Dyscontrol Scale as well as life adjustment problems, but get fairly low scores on measures of violence and sex drive. It thus seems reasonable to conclude that temporal lobe or any other form of epilepsy is not generally associated with violent behavior (although exceptions may exist). At the same time, we may conclude that if violence is associated with brain dysfunction, it is a type of dysfunction which is not usually described as epilepsy.

We should like to suggest that the Monroe Dyscontrol Scale holds promise of providing an index of brain dysfunction associated with epilepsy. Those patients with medically defined cases of epilepsy had significantly higher scores on the Monroe Scale than did other individuals. The scale is therefore one of the few noncognitive measures that reflect brain dysfunction. The dysfunction which is identified is related to affects and behaviors rather than to intellectual functioning. The scale provides a major new research tool that can be used to supplement the various batteries designed to measure organicity that are currently in use.

It is interesting that in addition to the self-referred violent individuals, male and female prisoners tend to get high scores on the violence measure, the psychopathic scale, and the scale designed to measure episodic dyscontrol. Individuals who show much overt violence therefore tend to have poor control. However, the converse is not true. Those individuals with high scores on episodic dyscontrol (e.g., epileptics) do not necessarily get high scores on the violence index.

These observations suggest that there may be a profile that will roughly describe individuals who show repeated acts of violence against other individuals. Such persons have a life history and life style which can be described in terms of a number of variables, variables which have been found to correlate with the presence of violence in most of the groups studied. The most important of these variables are a history of family violence, a tendency toward episodic dyscontrol states, a large number of life adjustment problems, behavior problems in family members, and certain schizoid or psychopathic tendencies. These variables can theoretically be combined into a multiple regression equation to predict the probability with which an individual will act violently.

In conclusion, we have proposed a methodology which we feel has great promise in helping us understand the nature of violent behavior shown by individuals. We have reported some tentative, preliminary findings which provide interesting hypotheses for future research. And finally, we have provided a set of psychometric tools which we feel will be of value in screening and research.

REFERENCES

Climent, C.E., Rollins, A., Ervin, R.F., and Plutchik, R. Epidemiological studies of women prisoners. I. Medical and psychiatric variables related to violent behavior. *American Journal of Psychiatry*, 1973, *130*, 985-990.

Coursin, D.B. Nutrition and brain function. In *Modern Nutrition in Health and Disease*, ed. M.G. Wohl and R.S. Goodhart. Philadelphia: Lea and Febiger, 1968.

Delgado, J.M.R. Aggressive behavior evoked by radio stimulation in monkey colonies. *American Zoologist*, 1966, *6*, 669-681.

Kellerman, H. The development of a forced-choice personality index and its relation to degree of maladjustment. Ph.D. Dissertation, Yeshiva University, 1964.

Mark, V.H., and Ervin, F.R. *Violence and the Brain*. New York: Harper & Row, 1970.

Monroe, R.R. *Episodic Behavioral Disorders*. Cambridge, Mass.: Harvard University Press, 1970.

Mooney, R.L. and Gordon L.V. *The Mooney Problem Checklist Manual*. New York: The Psychological Corp., 1950.

Mulvihill, D.J., and Tumin, M.M. *Crimes of Violence*. Report of National Commission on the Causes and Prevention of Violence, Washington, D.C., U.S. Government Printing Office, 1969.

Plutchik, R. *The emotions: facts, theories and a new model*. New York: Random House, 1962.

Plutchik, R. Emotions, evolution, and adaptive processes. In *Feelings and Emotions: The Loyola Symposium*, ed. M. Arnold. New York: Academic Press, 1970.

Plutchik, R. Problems of multidimensional evaluation. *Annals of the New York Academy of Sciences*, 1973, *218*, 78-86.

Plutchik, R., and Kellerman, H. *Manual for the Emotions Profile Index*. Los Angeles: Western Psychological Services, 1974.

Plutchik, R., Platman, S.R., Tilles, R., and Fieve, R.R. Construction and evaluation of a test for measuring mania and depression. *Journal of Clinical Psychology*, 1970, *26*, 499-503.

Roberts, W.W., and Kiess, H.O. Motivational properties of hypothalamic aggression in cats. *Journal of Comparative and Physiological Psychology*, 1964, *58*, 187-193.

Wasman, M., and Flynn, J.P. Directed attack elicited from the hypothalamus. *Archives of Neurology*, 1962, *6*, 220-227.

Wolfgang, M.E. *Patterns in Criminal Homicide.* Philadelphia: University of Pennsylvania Press, 1958.

Legal Implications of Psychosurgery

ROGER F. JOHNSON, M.D.
Johnson and Mahoney, P.C.
Denver, Colorado

A one-million-dollar lawsuit against three doctors and two hospitals in Detroit, Michigan, was reported in the *Denver Post* on Wednesday, January 9, 1974. It was alleged that the physicians and the hospitals had conspired to perform unneeded experimental brain surgery on a sixty-year-old former tool and die maker, who had previously suffered from epilepsy and mental illness. The complaint charged that

(1) The physicians had failed to properly inform the plaintiff of the nature of the experimental surgery; and

(2) That had the patient and/or his family been told of the experimental nature and possible consequences of the surgery, there would have been no need for the surgery, and the same would have been rejected.

The damages were claimed on the basis that the surgery, which involved the insertion of electrodes into the frontal lobes of the brain in an effort to destroy certain brain cells believed to have been causing abnormal, aggressive behavior, caused a worsening in the plaintiff's condition, requiring his permanent institutionalization.

In *Kaimowitz and John Doe* v. *Department of Mental Health for the State of Michigan, et al.*, Civil Action No. 73-19434-AW (Michigan,

Wayne County Circuit Court, July 10, 1973), a Michigan trial court ruled that an adult mental patient involuntarily detained in a mental institution cannot give legal, adequate consent to experimental brain surgery to relieve his uncontrollable aggression. Noting society's concern about violence and not desiring to impede medical progress, the court ruled, nonetheless, that psychosurgery could not be undertaken on involuntarily detained persons. The Court concluded that there was no scientific basis for saying that removal of a portion of the limbic brain would have any direct therapeutic effect.

In the *Tulane Law Review* in 1967, Howard Newcomb Morse reports that

> the lack of effective legal protection against a lobotomy being performed on a hospitalized mental patient is truly astounding. In Illinois, for example, as this writer has pointed out: "Once admitted, the person is at the mercy of the hospital Superintendant and Staff in that he may be subjected to a lobotomy . . . . " Under Article V of Section 5-5: " . . . Any patient hospitalized pursuant to the provisions of Article VI of this Act may be held under restraint and given treatment, *including surgery*." [Italicized portions were deleted from Illinois Act in 1965.]

He further points out:

> In respect to psychosurgery, . . . the Attorney General of Vermont rendered the following opinion:
>
> "As to the matter of securing the consent of the inmate's relatives, it is my belief that such is not necessary as a matter of law, but where it can be obtained, it is my feeling that such a course is one to be commended."

Serious legal questions are raised by these cases and comments and will be discussed in this paper.

1. The law of consent as it applies to an individual who
   (a) "Consents" to psychosurgery, or
   (b) Refuses psychosurgery.
2. The right of society to demand surgical intervention to alter behavior.
3. The liability of the surgeon doing experimental psychosurgery.
4. Recent efforts to regulate the doing of psychosurgery and trends in the law.
5. The distinction between *experimental* surgery (designed to get data only) and *innovative* surgery (new and unusual procedures designed as treatment with accumulation of data only a side benefit).

Psychosurgery has been meticulously defined by an Oregon statute as

> any operation or surgical procedure designed to irreversibly lesion or destroy brain tissue for the primary purpose of altering the thoughts,

> emotions, or behavior of a human being. Psychosurgery does not include procedures which may irreversibly lesion or destroy brain tissues when undertaken to cure well-defined disease states, such as brain tumor, epileptic foci, and certain chronic pain syndromes. (1 Oregon Revised Statutes, —, Sec. 677 —, Senate Bill No. 298, signed into law, June 1, 1973)

A review of the recent medical literature reveals there is no unanimity of opinion among scientific investigators as to the anticipated benefits and/or risks which might be expected in connection with psychosurgery.

Geschwind states in his note (*New England Journal of Medicine*, August 30, 1973, Vol. 289, No. 9): "The time is clearly appropriate for a careful, scientifically-controlled study of behavior-modifying surgery."

Kolb (*New England Journal of Medicine*, November 22, 1973, Vol. 289, No. 21) points out that the procedure is uncommon in this country: "Not a single psychosurgical procedure was carried out last year for patients with severe mental illness in the hospitals under the direction of the New York State Department of Mental Hygiene, the largest mental-hospital system in the country, if not the world."

Sweet has concluded (*New England Journal of Medicine*, November 22, 1973, Vol. 289, No. 21) that "the evidence now at hand indicates that those who have not responded to protracted intensive medical management should be appraised as possible candidates for surgery."

Graff, (*Journal of the American Medical Association*, January 28, 1974, Vol. 227, No. 4), states:

> Psychological and emotional consequences secondary to neurosurgical intervention in anybody's brain are quite likely. I can understand the use of neurosurgery for the treatment of anatomical and pathologic disorders for relief of conditions which are remediable by neurosurgical techniques. The limitations of the neurosurgeon with respect to treatment of patients with emotional disorders must be spelled out carefully.

Falconer said (*New England Journal of Medicine*, August 30, 1973, Vol. 289, No. 9): " . . . but there is as yet no evidence that the results of surgery by these methods [stereotactic measures to destroy selected targets] can compare with the more conventional methods that we have employed, and they usually fail to identify the pathological subtrait."

Betram Brown, Director of NIMH, said at the Kennedy hearings: "Not enough is known about the brain to support a clear justification for such operations."[1]

[1] *Science*, Vol. 179, March 16, 1973.

This scientific uncertainty has not escaped the attention of legal scholars.

Commenting on the involuntary treatment of mentally ill, Michael A. Peszke, M.D., states (*Connecticut Bar Journal,* Vol. 46, 1972), "*Involuntary Treatment of the Mentally Ill,*" that the arguments against the practice of involuntary psychiatric treatment are broken down into three criticisms:

(1) The medical model used to justify such treatment is not compatible with the realities of mental illness nor does it explain sufficiently the different life styles adopted by certain people.

(2) Involuntary treatment violates constitutional safeguards.

(3) People should have a right to treatment, and the commitment to a state psychiatric facility inevitably precludes that possibility.

The basic problem of nontherapeutic human experimentation is raised in a comment in the *Syracuse Law Review,* Vol. 24, 1067, 1973, entitled "*Non-Therapeutic Medical Research Involving Human Subjects.*" There it is pointed out that the experimental science of medicine has its origins prior to 200 A.D., but nonetheless, public awareness of the ethical and legal responsibilities posed by nontherapeutic human research did not become coalased until the Nuremberg War Trials.

The subject of experimental medicine and surgery has come to the attention of the Courts in numerous cases. The early case of *Carpenter* v. *Blake,* 60 Barb. 488, 514 York Supp. Court (1871), held that physicians must employ treatment methods which conform to established procedures, and a physician who engages in experimentation does so at his own peril.

Beginning in the 1930's however, we found a growing recognition of society's need for medical advance. In *Fortner* v. *Coke,* 272 Mich. 273, 261 NW 762 (1935), the Supreme Court of Michigan stated: "If the general practice of medicine and surgery is to progress, there must be a certain amount of experimentation carried on; but such experiments must be done with the knowledge and consent of the patient or those responsible for him, *and must not vary too radically from the accepted method of procedure*" (Emphasis added).

The Colorado Supreme Court considered experimental treatment in the case of *Jackson* v. *Burnham,* 20 Colo. 39, (1895). The Court instructed the jury as follows: "If you find from the evidence that this defendant, in the treatment of the plaintiff, omitted the ordinary or established mode of treatment, and pursued one that has proved injurious, it is of no consequence how much skill he may have; he has demonstrated a want of it in the treatment of the particular case, and is liable in damages."

To determine what is the proper test for proper treatment, the court stated, at pages 540-541:

> There must be some criterion in which to test the proper mode of treatment in a given case, and when a particular mode of treatment is upheld by a consensus of opinion among the members of the profession, it should be followed by the ordinary practitioner; and if a physician sees fit to experiment with some other mode, he should do so at his peril. In other words, he must be able, in the case of deleterious results, to satisfy the jury that he had reason for the faith that was in him, and justify his experiment by some reasonable theory.

The Court quotes from *Carpenter* v. *Blake, supra*:

> "Some standard, by which to determine the propriety of treatment, must be adopted; otherwise, experiment will take the place of skill, and the reckless experimentalist the place of the educated, experienced practitioner. . . . But when the case is one as to which a system of treatment has been followed for a long time, there should be no departure from it, unless the surgeon who does it is prepared to take the risk of establishing, by his success, the propriety and safety of his experiment."

> "The rule protects the community against reckless experiments, while it admits the adoption of new remedies and modes of treatment only when their benefits have been demonstrated, or when, from the necessity of the case, the surgeon or physician must be left to the exercise of his own skill and experience."

In reviewing the legal literature, one finds that there is a paucity of case law available on human experimentation. But certainly the ordinary rules of tort law would apply.

It is axiomatic, under our legal system, that elective surgery can be done only with the consent of the patient. The tort of battery is designed to protect the individual's interest in being free from intentional, unpermitted touchings of his person. Consent thus becomes a defense to an action for battery. In medical affairs, most of the states have held that a consent, in order to be effective, must be *an informed consent*. An informed consent entails an explanation of the ailment sought to be relieved, the procedure that was designed to afford the relief, and the substantial risks, if any, reasonably anticipated by the surgeon. Consent, in order to be effective, must also be voluntary, and voluntariness implies freedom to chose with reasonable comprehension from the available alternatives. Thus the potential subject of an experiment should be informed as to the nature of the experiment, direct and collateral hazards attending his participation, and all other information which may prove relevant to a decision to participate or not in the study. Many states hold that the extent of the disclosure should be measured by the yardstick of what other physicians would have disclosed under similar conditions.

In the recent case of *Canterbury* v. *Spence*, (D.C. Cir. 1972), 464 F. 2d 772, a different conclusion was reached.

A nineteen-year-old male patient was diagnosed as having sustained a rupture to an intervertebral disc. His surgeon advised that he undergo a laminectomy. When asked if the operation was serious, the doctor replied: "Not any more than any other operation." He did not further elaborate on any risks that were inherent in the procedure. Approximately one day after surgery the young man fell out of bed, and as a consequence was rendered paraplegic. In the ensuing litigation, it was alleged, among other things, that the surgeon had violated his responsibilities to the patient to adequately inform him of the risks.

In reversing a judgment of the lower court, the circuit court held: "The physician's duty to disclose is governed by the same legal principles applicable to others in comparable situations, with modifications only to the extent that medical judgment enters the picture. *We hold that the standard measuring performance of that duty by physicians, as by others, is conduct which is reasonable under the circumstances*" (Emphasis added).

The scope of the disclosure has been commented on by many courts. Various courts have adopted "medical custom," "good medical practice," "what a reasonable practitioner would have done under the circumstances," and others. In *Canterbury, supra*, it is stated:

> In our view, the patient's right of self decision shapes the boundaries of the duty to reveal. That right can be effectively exercised only if the patient possesses enough information to enable an intelligent choice. The scope of the physician's communications to the patient, then, must be measured by the patient's need, and that need is the information material to the decision. Thus, the test for determining whether a particular peril must be divulged is its materiality to the patient's decision: all risks potentially effecting the decision must be unmasked. As to safeguard the patient's interest in achieving his own determination and treatment, the law itself must set the standard for adequate disclosure.

It is pointed out that the physician stands in a fiduciary relationship to his patient and that the ordinary rules relating to fiduciaries will apply.

Aside from the ethical and moral considerations in the Declaration of Helsinki and the Nuremberg Code, the issue of consent becomes of primary legal importance in psychosurgery.

In *Kaimowitz and John Doe* v. *Department of Mental Health for the State of Michigan, et al., supra*, it appears that John Doe (whose real name is Louis Smith) was committed by the Kalamazoo County Circuit Court on January 11, 1955, to the Ionia State Hospital as a criminal sexual psychopath. He had been charged with the murder and rape of a student nurse at the Kalamazoo State Hospital while he was confined there as a mental patient. In 1972, Drs. Ernst Rodin and Jacques Gottlieb, of the Lafayette Clinic, a facility of the Michigan Department of Mental Health, proposed a study for the treatment of uncontrollable aggression. It was intended from such study to compare the effects of surgery on the amygdaloid portion of the limbic system of the brain with the effect of the drug cyproterone acetate on the male hormone flow. The experiment was intended to show which, if either, could be used in controlling aggression of males in an institutional setting and to afford lasting permanent relief from such aggression. After a search, John Doe was found to be the only appropriate candidate in the state mental system for such surgical experiment. Thereafter, John Doe and his parents signed an "informed consent" for John to become the experimental subject. The "informed consent" form provided in some detail what the proposed surgery was and what the proposed goals were. The risks were described as being "slight" but "could be potentially serious." These risks were stated to include infection, bleeding, temporary or permanent weakness or paralysis of one or more "of the legs or arms, difficulties with speech and thinking, as well as the ability to feel, touch, pain and temperature." Under extraordinary circumstances, it is also possible "that I might not survive the operation." Two separate three-man review committees were established by Dr. Rodin to review the scientific worthiness of the study and the validity of the consent form obtained from John Doe. Both committees approved the procedure and both gave their consent to such procedure. The surgery was scheduled for January 15, 1973, but shortly before that time, the plaintiff, Kaimowitz, a lawyer, became aware of the proposed experimental surgery on John Doe and made his concern known to the newspapers. Considerable publicity followed, and subsequently funds for the research project were stopped, and the experiment was canceled. Thereafter, the trial court ruled that the case should proceed on two issues framed as a Declaratory Judgment action. The two issues were as follows:

> (1) After failure of established therapies, may an adult, or a legally appointed guardian, if the adult is involuntarily detained at a facility within the jurisdiction of the State Department of Mental Health, give legally adequate consent to an innovative or experimental surgical procedure on the brain, if there is demonstrable, physical abnormality of the brain, and the procedure is designed to ameliorate behavior, which is either personally tormenting to the patient or so profoundly disruptive that the patient cannot safely live, or live with others?
> (2) If the answer to the above is yes, then is it legal in this state to undertake such innovative or experimental surgical procedure on the brain of

> an adult who is involuntarily detained at the facility within the jurisdiction of the State Department of Mental Health. . . .

The term "psychosurgery" was used by the court to describe the proposed innovative or experimental surgical procedure. In the definition of psychosurgery used there, it was essentially the same as described in this paper.

From the beginning of the trial, it was clear to the court from the testimony of witnesses that the understanding of the limbic system of the brain and its function is very limited. The record in that case was further demonstrative that animal experimentation in nonintrusive human experimentation had not been exhausted in determining brain function.

The court stated that

> violent behavior not associated with brain disease should not be dealt with surgically. At best, neurosurgery rightfully should concern itself with medical problems and not the behavior problems of a socio-ideology. The Court does not in any way desire to impede medical progress. We are much concerned with violence and the possible effects of brain disease on violence. Much research on the brain is necessary and must be carried on, but when it takes the form of psychosurgery, it cannot be undertaken on involuntarily detained populations. Other avenues of research must be utilized and developed.

The evidence showed that psychosurgery is clearly experimental, poses substantial danger to research subjects, and carries substantial unknown risks. All witnesses to the proceeding agreed that dangers were involved and the benefits to the patient were uncertain. Undesirable side-effects were described as flattening of emotional responses, decrease in the ability to reason abstractly, loss of capacity for new learning, and general sedation and apathy. Impairments in memory and unexpected responses to psychosurgery had been observed. "It was unanimously agreed by all witnesses that psychosurgery does not, given the present state of the art, provide any assurance that a dangerously violent person can be restored to the community."

The court concluded that *"We do hold that informed consent cannot be given by an involuntarily detained mental patient for experimental psychosurgery. . . ."* (Emphasis added).

The court notes that in order for a consent to be an effective and informed consent it must be *competent, knowing,* and *voluntary.* Commenting on the competency, the court points out that although the involuntarily detained patient may have sufficient I.Q. to comprehend his circumstances, "the very nature of his incarceration diminishes the capacity to consent to psychosurgery. The institutionalization tends to strip the individual of the support which will permit him to maintain his sense of self-worth and the value of his own physical and mental integrity. An involuntarily confined mental patient clearly has diminished capacity for making a decision about irreversible experimental psychosurgery."

The court further announced the rule that a guardian or a parent cannot do that which the patient, absent a guardian, would be legally unable to do.

Knowledge of the risk was in great question. From the evidence, it was clear that the facts surrounding experimental brain surgery were uncertain and the lack of knowledge on the subject made a knowledgeable consent to psychosurgery literally impossible.

And, as to the third element, voluntariness, the court concluded that involuntarily hospitalized patients are "not able to voluntarily give informed consent because of the inherent inequality of their position."

Although not necessary to the decision of the court, the court went on to consider three constitutional concerns.

The first consideration was that of the First Amendment.

> A person's mental processes, the communication of ideas, and the generation of ideas, come within the ambit of the First Amendment. The extent that the First Amendment protects the dissemination of ideas and the expression of thoughts, it equally must protect the individual's right to generate ideas. . . . Freedom of speech and expression, and the right of all men to disseminate ideas, popular or unpopular, are fundamental to ordered liberty. Government has no power or right to control men's minds, thoughts, and expressions. . . ."

The second constitutional concept involves the *right of privacy.* This concept basically relies upon the First, Fifth, and Fourteenth Amendments. The Ninth Circuit Court in *Mackey* v. *Procunier,* 477 F. 2d 877, 9th Cir. Ct., April 16, 1973, in reversing a District Court decision involving a prison inmate who had been subjected to shock treatments and experimental drug usage without his consent, stated: "Proof of such matters could, in our judgment, raise serious constitutional questions respecting cruel and unusual punishment or impermissible tinkering with the mental processes."

Intrusion into one's intellect, when one is involuntarily detained and subject to the control of institutional authorities, is an intrusion into one's constitutionally protected right of privacy.

The third and final constitutional protection is bottomed on violations of the Eighth Amendment against cruel and unusual punishment, the court here concluding that barring psychosurgery on this basis was a persuasive argument.

The court emphasized in its conclusion that when psychosurgery became an *accepted* neurosurgical procedure and was *no longer experimental*, that it would be possible *with appropriate review mechanism safeguards* that involuntarily detained mental patients could consent to an operation and that an involuntarily detained mental patient could give consent to an accepted neurosurgical procedure.

Other Courts have considered the problem. In the case of *Strunk* v. *Strunk*, 445 SW 2d 145 (Ky. 1969), the mother of an incompetent adult petitioned the Court for an Order authorizing the removal of a kidney from the incompetent adult for the purpose of transplanting the kidney into the body of his brother, who was at that time dying of a fatal kidney disease. The court there found that the operation was necessary, and that under the peculiar circumstances of this case, it would not only be beneficial to the brother but also beneficial to the donor, because the donor was greatly dependent upon the brother, both emotionally and psychologically, and his well-being would be jeopardized more severely by the loss of his brother than by the removal of a kidney. The Department of Mental Health for the State filed a brief amicus curiae and also recommended that the order be entered. The court there noted that the right to act for the incompetent in all cases has become recognized in this country as the doctrine of substituted judgment and is broad enough not only to cover property but also to cover all matters touching on the well-being of the ward. The court did conclude that their ruling would not extend so far as to allow the petitioner to subject the incompetent to a serious surgical procedure unless his life would be put in jeopardy. By this somewhat circuitous reasoning, the court has neatly side-stepped the serious considerations which we have been discussing in the surgical area of psychosurgery. In an interesting dissenting opinion in the *Strunk* case, *supra*, Justice Steinfeld, acknowledging his indelible recollection of a government, which to the everlasting shame of its citizens, embarked on a program of genocide and experimentation on human bodies, could not join in the majority opinion. He follows the more restrictive rule in stating that he is "unwilling to hold that the gate should be opened to permit the removal of an organ from an incompetent for transplant, at least until such time as it is conclusively demonstrated that it will be of significant benefit to the incompetent. . . . To hold that committees, guardians or Courts have such awesome power even in the persuasive case before us, could establish legal precedent, the dire result of which I cannot fathom. . . . "

A distinction must now be noted between *experimental* surgery and *innovative* surgery. What has been said to this point deals largely with experimental (only) surgery, having as its purpose the collection of data. Innovative surgery, with appropriate safeguards (i.e., animal experimentation), must certainly be viewed differently. Thus one might expect that the majority conclusion in *Strunk, supra,* would have been different if it had been shown that renal transplantation was an experimental procedure.

Based on what has been said, the personal liability of the neurosurgeon doing experimental surgery should be apparent. If the holding in *Kaimowitz, supra,* should be followed by appellate courts in other jurisdictions, then any consent obtained on the involuntarily hospitalized patient for experimental surgery would be ineffective, and the surgeon who performed such surgery could be liable for assault and battery. For this, his insurance company could be called upon to pay damages. This in itself raises the interesting question as to whether the professional liability insurance policy would cover such a claim. Although the language in insurance policies may differ to some extent, in general, coverage is provided "to pay all loss by reason of the liability imposed by law upon the insured for damages on account of professional services rendered or which should have been rendered."

Some policies specifically exclude certain matters such as assault and battery, libel and slander, breach of contract, and other similar actions. If a surgeon were insured under a policy which excluded assault and battery, then he could find himself in a situation where his professional liability insurance was not available to either defend the action or pay damages.

In his book, *Private Conscience and Public Law,* New York: Fordham University Press, 1972, Richard J. Regan, S.J., points out "that claims of conscience may also run counter to the interests of state and local governments in the protection of public welfare, and prominent among such interests are those involving the health of citizens."

Claims of public health interest may also conflict with claims of individuals to bodily integrity. In *Jacobson* v. *Massachusetts,* 197 U.S. 11 (1905), Jacobson was convicted of refusal to submit himself to mandatory vaccination against smallpox. His conviction was sustained on appeal to the Supreme Court of the United States. His basic objection was not religious but rather that compulsory vaccination law was "unreasonable, arbitrary, oppressive and hostile to the inherent right of every free man to care for his own body and health in such a way as to him seems best and that the execution of such a law against one who objected to vaccination was an assault upon his person."

The United States Supreme Court overrode his objections and

pointed out that the community has a right to protect itself against the threat of an epidemic disease.

Compulsory sterilization was considered in the 1927 United States Supreme Court case of *Buck* v. *Bell*, 274 U.S. 200 (1927). In that case, lawyers for Carrie Buck, a feeble-minded patient in a state hospital, whose mother and illegitimate daughter were also feeble-minded, challenged a Virginia statute which provided for compulsory sterilization of institutionalized mental defectives. Justice Holmes upheld the law, stating: "The principle that sustains compulsory vaccination is broad enough to cover the cutting of the Fallopian tubes. . . . Three generations of imbeciles are enough."

It would appear, then, in conclusion, that there are really two broad areas of law which have been commented upon: the first involves the rights of the individual as a subject in experimental brain surgery, and the second involves the rights of society to impose such surgery on its members. A third area, as has been mentioned, involves the responsibilities of the surgeon performing such surgery, insofar as these surgical procedures may give rise to professional liability lawsuits.

A legal solution has been proposed in Oregon through the adoption of its statute regulating experimental psychosurgery. Other legal authors have proposed similar regulations in the form of committees composed of physicians, lawyers, and members of the community. Others have suggested the courts as the decision-making forum.[2] It will probably require the combined efforts of the courts, the legislatures, and the medical and legal professions if the orderly development of psychosurgery is to occur.

REFERENCES

Buck v. *Bell*, 274 U.S. 200 (1927).

Campbell, Horace E., "Editorial," *Rocky Mountain Medical Journal*, Vol. 71, No. 7.

Canterbury v. *Spence*, 464 F. 2d 772 (D.C. Cir. 1972).

Carpenter v. *Blake*, 60 Barb. 488, 514 York Supp. Court (1871).

Declaration of Helsinki.

Falconer, *New England Journal of Medicine*, Vol. 289, No. 9, August 30, 1973.

Fortner v. *Coke*, 272 Mich. 273, 261 NW 7.

Geschwind, *New England Journal of Medicine*, Vol. 289, No. 9, August 30, 1973.

Graff, *Journal of the American Medical Association*, Vol. 227, No. 4, January 28, 1974.

Jackson v. *Burnham*, 20 Colo. 39 (1895).

---

[2] Horace E. Campbell, Editorial, *Rocky Mountain Medical Journal*, July 1974, Vol. 71, No. 7.

Jacobson v. *Massachusetts,* 197 U.S. 11 (1905).

Kaimowitz and John Doe v. *Department of Mental Health for the State of Michigan,* No. 73-19434-AW (Michigan, Wayne County Circuit Court, July 10, 1973).

Kolb, *New England Journal of Medicine,* Vol. 289, No. 21, November 22, 1973.

Mackey v. *Procunier,* 477 F. 2d 877, 9th Cir. Ct., April 16, 1973.

Morse, Howard Newcomb, *Tulane Law Review,* 1967.

Nuremberg Code

1 Oregon Revised Statutes, —, Sec. 677, Senate Bill No. 298, Signed into Law, June 1, 1973.

Peszke, Michael A., M.D., "Involuntary Treatment of the Mentally Ill," *Connecticut Bar Journal,* Vol. 46, 1972.

Regan, Richard J., S.J., *Private Conscience and Public Law,* New York: Fordham University Press, 1972.

Science, Vol. 179, March 16, 1973.

Strunk v. *Strunk,* 445 SW 2d 145 (Ky. 1969).

Sweet, *New England Journal of Medicine,* Vol. 289, No. 21, November 22, 1973.

Syracuse Law Review, "Non-Therapeutic Medical Research Involving Human Subjects," Vol. 24, 1967, 1973.

*Brain Control in a Democratic Society**

ROBERT J. GRIMM
Neurological Sciences Institute
Good Samaritan Hospital & Medical Center
Portland, Oregon

INTRODUCTION

Do not adjust your mind.
There is a fault in reality.

Written on an Oxford
University wall

there
is
absolutely
no
inevitability
as
long
as
there
is
a
willingness
to
contemplate
what
is
happening.

Marshall McLuhan

*Presented at the Fifth Annual Cerebral Function Symposium: Dyssocial Behavior Control and Cerebral Function, San Diego, California, March 8, 1974.

Ours may be the last generation to inquire openly about brain control of individuals by the state. An open inquiry means a searching and public appraisal of emerging control technology and its dangers to a democratic society. The weight of such an inquiry falls not upon methods, but upon the circumstances of control use. As fearful questions, simply put: Who will administer these controls and for what reason? Do I get them if I want them or not?

Brain control means the capture of those executive faculties of thought which direct and sustain our behavior. The method of capture is academic. Between the notions *state* and *individual* lie those essential transactions between a person and his country which deliver his security, his pleasures, and his agony.

I provide no distinction between new technologies of brain control and behavioral control. It would hardly matter to the person who knew that his life was being, or had been, arranged elsewhere. You may see as imprecise and inflammatory my labeling behavioral control "brain control." Why mince words? Reduction of conflict between an individual and the state, even where contracted freely, *is* brain control, however congenial it might appear to self-identified ends. Where this interaction occurs without knowledge or consent, it is devoid of ethical or constitutional standing. Where such controls are deep and pervasive, and are exercised to hold a person's life in escrow, distinctions between contracted and enforced control are meaningless. We focus here on the emergence of brain controls in America, present and potential antecedents for use of controls, and the sticky questions: Who will do what to whom, and why?

Four premises in our own times bear on the probable emergence of brain control within our society, a technocracy in transition, if not decline. They are unpleasant to think about and are therefore deserving of the widest and deepest public discussion. I shall state them briefly and return to examine each in some depth.

PREMISES

The first premise has to do with our unsettling times. Western technocracy is in transition, en route to what the distinguished Harvard economist Daniel Bell and others term a "post-industrial society" (Bell, 1973; Marien, 1973). It is a regressive transition. Arrival time to the roughest period of survival is predicted to be about the year 2000 A.D. or shortly thereafter. The economic, political, and environmental "storm of crises" (Platt, 1969) predicted will be increasingly painful for all. Hard times will require the rise of what Heilbroner (1974) terms an "iron government," an authoritarian state organized to keep us together as a nation. As an item of faith, such states will use what minimum controls are necessary to maintain order and promote tranquility.

The second premise is that brain control technology is advanced and increasingly sophisticated. It is being tested in this and other countries and will be available to the state as the need arises.

The third premise is that neuroscientists will be asked to provide and transcribe brain control techniques for the state and that they will "deliver" when asked.

The fourth premise is that physicians—and in particular psychiatrists—will become the principal agents of control; the argument here is that dissent or nonidentity with the needs of a beleaguered state will be viewed as mental illness requiring treatment. The task will be to change minds, not society.

Given these premises, we turn now to examine the evidence for each in turn.

AN IRON GOVERNMENT IN AMERICA

> It is not the consciousness of men that determines their existence, but on the contrary, it is their social existence that determines consciousness.
>
> Karl Marx

In his brilliant analysis of the antecedents of coming hard times in America, Heilbroner (1974) used the term "iron government." This speaks of a state organized in response to an expected breakdown in American society between now and the first decades of the twenty-first century. The smash-up is the end stage of a technology which provided two centuries of material wealth, but which has also failed to satisfy the human spirit.

In asking, "What is the human prospect?" Heilbroner reflected on the depressed mood of the country; those "confidence-shaking events" of the Vietnam war, street crime and assassinations, bizarre hijackings and kidnappings, the collapse of integrity in the Executive Branch, and so forth, that unveiled, as he put it, the "barbarisms behind the amenities of life." There were also the deeper disappointments: the failure to pass our values to our children; disappearance of the bonds of community; and loss of a collective social assurance that reforms in welfare, medical, and educational systems could be accomplished by the legislative process. And lastly, we now realize that environmental deterioration is directly linked with industrial growth.

Threading these disquieting themes runs a critical uneasiness, found in the writing of Marcuse (*One Dimensional Man*, 1964), Theodore Roszak (*The Making of the Counter Culture*, 1969; *Where the Wasteland Ends*, 1973), Reich (*The Greening of America*, 1970), and Keniston (*The Uncommitted: Alienated Youth in American Society*, 1965), and in the economic analyses of Galbraith (*The New Industrial State*, 1967) and Richard Goodwin (*New Yorker*, 1973), that a dehumanizing technostructure, powered up by its own logic, has fragmented and dried up human community in this culture. We live as aliens apart and indistinguishable except by machines of our own choosing.

Heilbroner passes next to the "external challenges" presaging the arrival of an iron government: the demographic crisis, an expotential population rise to more than 7 billion humans within thirty-three years, the doubling time at current world birth rates (Meadows et al, 1972); and a promise of threatened "wars of redistribution," whereby underdeveloped nations possessing the Bomb attempt nuclear blackmail, using it as a sword of Damocles to secure their own economic needs. The current politics of oil is perhaps a libretto of this dream. Lastly, there are the ecologic disturbances engendered by industrial growth, resource depletion and pollution.

The consequence of these external challenges, as suggested by a "world standard run" on the Club of Rome's computer (Meadows et al, 1972, p. 124, Fig. 35), is a profound leveling of wealth between rich and poor nations to assure spaceship earth's survival. It is this leveling that will, in this country, move us away from flexible alternatives in social structures (the "democratic") toward a more stable, *fixed* society, a more uniform, planned state. It is this compressing process that will call forth an iron government.

Such governments will undoubtedly have differences in makeup. In countries with explosive population growth unchecked by voluntary means, growth will be halted by more repressive measures. In the United States, an iron government will have to deal with a serious public response to the evolution of a static, no-growth economy—the conversion, as Kenneth Boulding put it, from a cowboy to a spaceman economy. A no-growth or stationary economy generates a crisis as a consequence of a significant and enforced income redestribution, an abolition of dreams tied to economic rewards, and an ending to the growth theory of capitalism and socialism alike. A totalitarian government is the unique survival response of a complex state attempting to head off disastrous social polarizations as amenities of life atrophy.

However we assess Heilbroner's sobering view, it does represent one respected economist's effort to think about his nation's course as its organization and world position falters. The measure and sobriety of his concern is reflected in a passage found toward the end of his essay:

> The search for scientific knowledge, the delight in intellectual heresy, the freedom to order one's life as one pleases are not likely to be easily contained within the tradition oriented, static society I have depicted. To a very great degree, the public must take precedence over the private—an aim which it is easy to give lip service in the abstract, but difficult for someone used to the pleasures of political, social, and intellectual freedom to accept in fact. (p. 34)

What are the steps between future shocks—today and tomorrow? How much time do we have, and how shall each of us fare? Beyond issues of data banks, privacy, credit cards and other technologic imperatives, whatever the path, it can be predicted that the notion of an individual as a person will disappear, the victim of what Galbraith (1968) has termed the "principle of consistency." Individuals today are increasingly identified as to their job or function, not for their personal uniqueness. The consistency principle asserts the extreme interdependence of people, organizations, and the state. It is the consistency of functions that link wages and services, the consistency of narrowed specialization and the consistency of purpose, institutions and bee colonies alike. The individual gradually becomes a function for assignment. The term "individualism" will be transcribed as *dysfunction* if not *dissent*.

As boundaries of a stationary economy become clear and our roles more proscribed, drastic, if not unpredictable alterations can be expected in myths of personal identity. Here lies the genesis of serious and practical conflicts: conflicts over resources, living space, family size, income, privacy, and power. It is the predicted magnitude of such conflicts that will call out a stabilizing state, however "iron" in its makeup.

But let us be more precise. What is the iron government and what does it want? Do we have any clues as to its nature other than Heilbronner's guess that it will be a mix of socialism and militarism? Are we talking of a *Brave New World* or *1984*? It is doubtful that such dystopias are in the immediate future or that more vulgar and totalitarian models will obtain, at least in the United States. An iron government essentially will mean something powerful, but one quite likely benign and indifferent in its external appearance. I imagine it to be an extension of many things we live with today. It will be an assembly logic of millions of people-functions: a colony of functions tightly planned and more integrated, a system whirring away, a social automaton. Another view of the iron government as a function is to picture a magnificent watch with built-in positive and negative feed-back control loops to monitor, induce, and realign cooperation between its many functions (parts, people) necessary to the logic and synchrony of its programs, if not its survival.

There are two models which exist today that give a taste of such future iron governments. The first is an efficient bureaucracy. The second is the problem of "women and madness" (Chesler, 1972). The first is of interest not as an object lesson of a whirring system of specialized human functions geared to a purpose, but for the question of how a bureaucracy deals with individualism—i.e., dissent. The second example concerning women is the problem of defining roles in such a way that dissent or straying too far from an assigned role can eventually be viewed as either dissent or insanity, arguments that have come out of the women's liberation movement. We look first at the way a bureaucracy deals with dissent.

In a discussion of the exercise of subtle and efficient control over individual behavior, Goodwin (1974, III) provides a glimpse of the power and purpose of organizations:

> The interest—the intrinsic purpose—of modern economic structure is not simply the accumulation of wealth; its manner and scale of operation are ends in themselves. Because control adequate to guarantee this function—to protect against all present conflict and future change—is a mirage, the impulse toward control is insatiable. It directs a continuing attack on all authority that is independent of the economic structure: not just on state or legal authority but on alternative repositories of social power—principally on forms of social cohesion *which might give expression to human wants inconsistent with the present structure of society.* [italics mine]

And the paragraph that follows:

> The bureaucratic danger to liberty does not take the form of direct and overt repression by government. It manifests itself in subtler means of coercion—a system of rewards and penalties which dulls the urge toward individual expression and makes the inability to exercise liberty appear a consequence of individual and institutional choice.

For women, Phyllis Chesler (1972) argues that they have already arrived at the point where they are viewed as a collage of functions and that disagreement or incongruity with these essentially male-proscribed roles is viewed as madness or insanity. If it's bad enough, it is treated, and this includes institutionalization.

In suggesting that as our technocracy winds down in response to imposed external and internal forces, the argument is that this will cause enough social conflict to necessitate the rise of a stabilizing iron government, here given a functional interpretation, a super-program to plan and synchronize life. It boils down to the conclusion that individual uniqueness will disappear, replaced by trained, sorted, and assigned functions, one set to the citizen. The iron government is the plan and context for survival in a troubled world. Where dissonance occurs with respect to the state, it will require for survival—impossible outside of the system—controls upon a citizen's life or thought.

BRAIN CONTROL TECHNOLOGY

For both caretakers and subjects (Romano-V., 1974), it becomes clear that an authoritarian state will need to control behavior. This is to insure the operation of the system, as well as to manage those who are either not needed or are dissidents. Reliable, inexpensive controls applicable to all without detectable intellectual impairment (the cost-benefit ratio problem)—this is a useful prescription. If voluntary use of such controls could be provided as positive reinforcement by the state, and anxiety over control extinguished, such brain control would be indistinguishable from the identity and function of the state, which brings us to the second premise: brain control technology is moderately advanced, is being tested under various circumstances, and will be available to the state as the need arises.

Before inquiring about the state of the art, a word about the perceived discomfort of those of us who work on such controls or debate their use.

We enter an era of profound interest in the brain. It is a period in which sooner or later we shall begin a debate more profound and certainly wider than that which arose between nuclear physicists over the issue of the Bomb after Hiroshima.[1] Do scientists have the right to pursue projects potentially destructive of human life, and in this era, destructive of the individual? Such moral issues were repeatedly raised during the Vietnam war over issues of weapon development, germ warfare, and massive forest defoliation. They surface now over the issue of psychosurgery and technical efforts to deal with aggression and dyssocial behavior. A chapter of the Society for Neuroscience recently called for a moratorium on psychosurgery not meeting standards to be set by a national commission (Burke et al, 1973).

[1]Nuclear physicists debated not only the issue of continuance of their work on such projects, but over the matter of civilian versus military control of the use of the Bomb, atomic energy, and later the building of the hydrogen bomb. The exploding of a nuclear device by the Russians on August 29, 1949, silenced the opposition. For an account of this struggle see Walter and Miriam Schneir's account of this period in *Invitation to an Inquest*, 1965.

Elsewhere, Oregon legislators passed a bill in 1973 requiring board review of all psychosurgery and electrical brain stimulation practice.[2] Neuroscientists will be under increasing pressure to examine their individual and collective position vis-à-vis the widening issue of brain control applications in a democratic society. We cannot escape this responsibility. Hopefully such examination shall proceed, untutored by the needs of the state, and in an atmosphere where our contribution of methodology productive of brain control can be argued fairly.

We can begin by asking about the current state of the art. What would a catalog of techniques contain? I shall review in a general way the more discussed methods, but will omit from the symposium manuscript all citations describing techniques which seem to me immediately applicable to humans. Reluctance to do so is a measure of a deepening apprehension over the ethical matter of publically detailing or referencing methods which could be used to the detriment or control of another's behavior.[3]

Psychosurgery and Electrical Brain Stimulation

Of the brain control technologies available, it is dubious that either stereotaxic psychosurgery or chronic depth electrical brain stimulation (EBS) are of much use. Both approaches are expensive, imprecise, based on unsatisfactory data, are the treatment of choice of no recognized illness, and are absolutely unpredictable in outcome. This last fact certifies their experimental if not nonsurgical nature and makes it implausible that either can be covered by the canon of informed consent. There are enthusiasts of this procedure, but I believe their scientific and clinical positions to be unsound and ill-served by arguments defending a privilege of treatment contract with patients or

[2] In June, 1973, Senate Bill 298 was passed by the Oregon legislature and signed into law by Governor Thomas McCall. It provided for a Board of Review for psychosurgical procedures and the use of depth electrical brain stimulation designed to alter behavior. Electroconvulsive therapy (ECT) was specifically excluded, as it would have engendered the defeat of the bill by psychiatrists, who use shock treatment as therapy. For a background of the legislative effort, see Grimm (1973), and for a more general account of the circumstances of the bill's writing and passage, see Dow, Grimm, and Rushmer.

[3] How journal editors might respond to papers submitted lacking a *Methods* section is unknown. There are precedents, however, for withholding information detrimental to endangered species. It is customary, for example, in field-study literature dealing with the prarie falcon (*Falco mexicanus*) to omit the nest site location to preclude human predation. The same practice is followed by mushroomers when asked to provide maps to the location of the more edible morels (e.g., *Morchella esculenta*) or polypores (e.g., *Polyporous sulphureus*).

the position that without such efforts, advancement in the science of brain function will falter, or that legislative attack on psychosurgery per se provides an opening wedge for federal involvement in research.

Let me pinpoint some specific psychosurgery procedures to suggest that they are unimportant clinically. Stereotaxic lesions have been advocated for the management of the aggressive individual with or without a seizure disorder (Mark and Ervin, 1970); obsessive compulsive neuroses (Meyer et al, 1973); pederast homosexuality (Roeder et al, 1972); aggressive, hyperkinetic children (Andy and Jurko, 1972); addiction syndromes (Knight, 1966), and cancer pain (Laitinen and Vilkki, 1972).

Aggression and various forms of dyssocial behavior have been a source of considerable concern in the last decade.[4] In terms of psychosurgical procedures, two kinds of aggressive or criminally assaultive patients have been described, those with and without temporal lobe epilepsy (TLE). But both have been viewed as potential candidates for amygdala lesions. The argument in the TLE patient is that paroxysmal bursts disorganize the activities of the amygdala nuclear complex, re-

[4]The National Institute of Neurologic Diseases and Stroke committee summary (Goldstein, 1974) is neither a critical review of literature cited or a complete review of pertinent literature; 588 entries are listed in the bibliography, 388 of which pertain to animal studies. A cross-check of the 388 entries with the bibliography of Clemente and Chase ("Neurological substrates of aggressive behavior," *Ann. Rev. Physiol.* 35:329-356) and the Avis review ("The neuropharmacology of aggression," 1973) shows that the NINDS work (covering the same period) contains approximately 50% or fewer of research papers pertinent to the subject; the overlap between these three reviews of the same subject is small. The readings which present broader perspectives of aggression in man included Konrad Lorenz's *On Aggression* (1966), Robert Ardrey's *Territorial Imperative* (1966), A.H. Buss's *The Psychology of Aggression* (1961), and the views of two analytically trained humanists, Eric Fromm's *The Anatomy of Destructiveness* (1973) and Silvano Arieti's *The Will to be Human* (1972). Valenstein's book (1973) is the most thorough review of the background of psychosurgery. Smith's discussion of the aggressive potential of amphetamines (missing from the NINDS review) is quite useful ("Speed freaks versus acid heads: conflict between drug subcultures," *Clin. Peds.* 2:185-192, 1969). The omission in the NINDS review of any reference to Peter Breggin's writing or the recent Detroit legal case having to do with psychosurgery (Kaimowitz, Doe, et al, 1973; Rodin, AC exhibits, 1973) or other political issues that have intruded into sanctioning brain control procedures on aggressive individuals is understandable but lamentable. The public and scientific debate over the issue of psychosurgery cannot be placed in historical context without reference at least to Breggin's *Congressional Record* reviews (1972a,b) or to the letter "Role of brain disease in riots and urban violence" published in the *Journal of the American Medical Association* 201:895 (1967) by Drs. Mark, Sweet, and Ervin. Vernon Mark's "Brain surgery in aggressive epileptics" should be required reading of all those who would cast stones (*Hastings Center Report* 3:1-5, 1973).

sulting in rage episodes. All observers agree that if this does occur among TLE patients, it is extremely rare and the rage seen may be independent of the paroxysmal disorder. Amygdalotomies in such patients have no predictable effect on either seizure frequency or form, may do nothing with the rage, and are not innocuous either to intellectual or behavioral effects (Valenstein, 1973; Goldstein, 1974; Horowitz, 1970).

The question of performing amygdalotomies on patients without evidence of limbic lobe paroxysmal discharges basically deals with more philosophic questions about psychosurgery, and the dimensions of one's cultural understanding of or sensitivity to the origins of violence. As episodic dyscontrol syndromes (Bach y Rita et al, 1971) are not correlated with EEG evidence of paroxysmal disorders of the temporal lobe or limbic system, the question of amygdalotomy for brain control of such aggression is one that holds little interest for most physicians. Such procedures are now being argued in the courts and legislatures, and support seems difficult to muster.

Cutting the cingulum pathway to reduce chronic anxiety or compulsions is not unlike dealing with double vision by optic nerve section. Hypothalamic lesions for homosexuals may or may not be due to chemical castration, but as the current controversy of whether or not homosexuality is a disease or a variation in life styles leaves little support for either this procedure or the bizarre therapy of thalamotomy for restless, disordered children. As for addiction syndromes, even in the hands of Walter Freeman, who made very large lesions, the procedures were unpredictable and ill-advised (1959). Finally, cingulotomies for control of cancer pain are last resorts. They may work but do not affect pain, only its affective response. The procedure is not predictable in its outcome (J. Seres, personal communication).

> Ninety-nine percent of the recruits were given amnesia upon arriving on Mars. Their memories were cleaned out by mental health experts, and Martian surgeons installed radio antennas in their skulls in order that recruits might be radio controlled.
>
> —Kurt Vonnegut, Jr.,
> *The Sirens of Titan* (1959)

Depth stimulation electrode techniques are extremely sophisticated in animal experiments. They can be remotely controlled, information either sent or received by telemetering devices within the skull to release electrical or chemical stimuli. Programs can be devised to reward, punish, or blank neural operations and their behavioral concomitants. But such techniques are extraordinarily dangerous. When applied to the alert human, to an electrically evoked movement of the hand or a verbal phrase or sound, all subjects reply, when asked why they did what they did, that they wanted to do it; that the will to perform the movement came from them. Use of EBS by telemetered control in the immediate future is unlikely for practical reasons. The use of devices to locate the whereabouts of paroles implanted with signal sources is another matter touching on control but beyond the limits of this discussion.

Psychopharmacologic Agents: A Trojan Horse

> Changing the human environment is a monumental undertaking. While seeking to change cognitive shapes through chemical means is more convenient and economical, the drug solution has already become another Trojan horse.
>
> —Leonard et al. (1970)

What are we to make of the drug revolution in the United States? As a people, we annually use huge quantities of alcohol, tobacco, coffee, cannabis, and psychotropic drugs to alter our experience, and modify anxiety, insomnia, depression, hallucinatory and manic periods. Is it true, as Weil (1973) asserts, that "the desire to alter consciousness periodically is an innate, normal desire analogous to hunger or sexual drive" (p. 19)? The 1974 *Physicians' Desk Reference* lists sixty companies which compound more than 225 psychopharmacologic preparations embracing thirty-five to forty different chemicals, depending upon what you count. They serve as sedatives, hypnotics, tranquilizers, antidepressants, and antipsychotics. Two of the three most prescribed drugs in the United States today are tranquilizers (Klerman, 1972; Ferguson, 1973). Estimates vary, but perhaps 50% of our current population take one of these drugs infrequently; 17% use psychotropics regularly and most adults use others—e.g., coffee, amphetamines, marijuana, tobacco. We live in a culture where drugs are used widely and accepted for their power to modify or extend experience, or subdue conflict. This being so, drugs may assist in furthering the aims of the state, as they are predicted to become more effective and precise in their actions, and less toxic. A drug to eliminate anger or promote acceptance without touching other activities of mind would be of significance to a totalitarian state.

Three drug issues bear on the question of availability and practice of control. The first is the physician-patient relationship. A common strategy with patients in trouble, major or minor, is to change minds and not environments—to use a drug that will move up or down the threshold for dealing with their lives. The assumption here is that when a depression is lifted or anxiety quieted one of two things happens: improved "accommodation" to the system occurs, or a more benign, if not realistic, acceptance of a personal fate is achieved. Medicine is the agency of control, drawing legitimacy from the physician's role as healer, and it does not correct or challenge social, economic, or political environments which may have set up the conflict. Where drug use leads to iatrogenic illness, including addiction, the medical issues provide a treatable organic condition, twice removed from its environmental trigger. We have conditioned ourselves to the easier task of altering minds to fit environments; this has increased our vulnerability to control and also focuses attention on the role of the physician.

A second issue provides an example of drug use for a specific but complex purpose—education—in a population of prepubertal children. This is the practice of prescribing amphetamines and their analogue methylphenidate hydrochloride (Ritalin) for restless, disruptive boys or children diagnosed as having minimal brain dysfunction (MBD) with or without learning problems (Clements, 1966). Children with this syndrome may respond dramatically to small, routine dosages of such medicines for a period of time. There are now approximately one-quarter of a million American children on these drugs, and questions are being raised not only about the long-term effects of the drugs, but also about their "political" use. Is it an interesting brain control experiment in America, or is it sound clinical medicine mixing together, as it does, bits of behavior, learning, growth, the classroom, and drugs prescribed by the physician?

First, there is the problem that it is boys who are the main drug target. A good clinical rule is that if a boy is brought to the physician by parents at the request of the school, until proven otherwise, look to the family for some unpleasant "hidden" agenda sponsoring the behavior. If it is a girl, sexism aside, the issue is usually more serious.

While there is little question that these drugs can change behavior of children with hyperkinesis, given strict adherence to diagnostic criteria (Grinspoon and Singer, 1973), are we basically using these drugs on children to "retool a normal personality variation to fit the school system?" (Steinfels, 1972). Are children being modified to better fit the normative operations of the public schoolroom, reducing not only their own dissonance but also providing the order necessary for the teacher to operate, others to learn, and a family to exercise its authority?

Without proof of an organic lesion in MBD children, and given the fact that amphetamines will alter behavior, this still is not evidence of imputed dysfunction. Curiously, there are few studies of long-term effects of these drugs on children. Indeed, the few that have been published are either uncontrolled, of short length, or are frankly worrisome, as the question recently raised about whether such drugs retard growth (Safer et al, 1972). The possibility has also been suggested that such treatment in children conditions them to drug use in later life (Ladd, 1970). As the long-term effects in children are unknown, the level of agreement promoted by drug houses among educators, physicians, and parents is worrisome, to say the least. It provides an example of a willingness to compress a quite possibly normal range of development to fit specific goals of a tightly organized system.

The charge made by the *Washington Post* on June 29, 1970 ("Omaha Pupils Given Behavior Drugs," 1970), was that 5% to 10% of Omaha, Nebraska, children were being given "behavioral modification drugs to improve classroom deportment and increase learning potential." (This was erroneous; the 5% to 10% figure was an estimate of the prevalence of learning disabilities of children in that school system.) Considerable publicity was given to the report (Hunsinger, 1970; Ladd, 1970) and a subsequent federal investigation was held to air the entire matter, underscoring a sensitive political issue ("Federal involvement . . ." 1970).

A third example of drug use for brain control involves obtaining behavioral changes in institutionalized patients or prisoners. Questions are being raised about institutionalization, drug use, and the "double-agent" role of the institution doctor in promoting the needs of the institution over the needs of the individual: are not drugs given to achieve institutional norms whether or not they have any resemblance to outer society? The suggestion is that they are, and in the double-agent role, the individual loses, the institution wins (Goffman, 1961; Halleck, 1971).

Drug use by prison inmates takes three forms. The first is the illicit use of drugs as heroin to escape the regressive features of prison life ("'H' on the campus? Prisoners do better, do their time, just lay back." Arthur Simmons, personal communication). A second use is to reduce anxiety, depression, and psychoses.[5] The third is use of drugs as agents of punishment or coercion—e.g., apomorphine (Fox et al, 1973), succinyl choline (worked out in alcoholics, Sanderson *et al*, 1964), and long-acting fluphenazines (Prolixin) to reduce aggressiveness, or as an adjunct to behavior modification.

Drug punishment of prisoners is a subject of some debate. But as it

[5] Therapeutic interruption of the process of vengeance is in the old tradition of seeing to the good health of the imprisoned criminal so that his terror (or torture) would not be mitigated. This was done so that punishment was given in equal measure to the distress of the victim. The relationship of this idea to insanity rules is discussed by Menninger (1968).

remains outside penal codes and legal decisions on prisoners' rights (Schwitzgebel, 1971; McGarry and Kaplan, 1973), and violates the Declaration of Helsinki (1964), the Nuremberg Code (1947), and the ethical principles of the American Medical Association (1957)—especially as recently restated by psychiatrists (1973)—it can scarcely receive support from ethical physicians.

Are we working out in many groups of this century the differential use of drugs for the twenty-first century? Is the phenomenal rise in use of marijuana as a consciousness expander a format for our transition to a new age? Certainly a drug that provides the illusion of peace and freedom—the vision of how things hoped for or should be—in the midst of a fragmented, technologic society with abundant misery must be terribly useful as a diversion and sanction for inactivity. The nasty thing here involves drug use certifying the contract of healing between a patient and his physician. It validates the principle of altering mind and not environment. Halleck (1971, p. 77) stated the dilemma well: "What will happen when a psychiatrist can cure a symptom without having to address its cause?" The present Drug Culture at all levels in American life emerges as a Trojan horse, a method of masking, subduing, and abolishing social discontent by aegis of the medical model.

> If Ritalin is good for an overactive child would it be good for a hyperkinetic country?
>
> —Peter Steinfels
> "Confronting the other drug problem" (1972)

> What if while they were in jail Henry David Thoreau, Eugene Debs, Martin Luther King, and Malcolm X had been given the opportunity to improve their mental outlook by taking a powerful antidepressant?
>
> —Seymour Halleck,
> *The Politics of Therapy* (1971)

The last control technology to be considered is the direct manipulation of behavior.

Adjusting Behavior

> We should reshape our society so that we all would be trained from birth to do what society wants us to do.
>
> —J.V. McConnel,
> *Psychology Today* (1970)

Behavioral modification technology and its utopian purposes are set forth in two of B.F. Skinner's books *Walden II* (originally published 1948) and *Beyond Freedom and Dignity* (1971). By altering our environment in explicit ways, Skinner argues that the inner, primitive "autonomous man"—one's chaos of uniqueness—can be shaped to make a better society. All that is needed are contingencies and reinforcements. Judging from the virtuoso performance of Skinner's critics,[6] we find another painful symptom of the recognition by a troubled conscience that he may be right—that contributions to the design of a more rational man can be made to bring more harmony with the state, which may well be beyond freedom and dignity. But is the price too high?

Behavior modification was originally a clinical matter. It focused on such problems as phobias, hysterical blindness, and autistic children (Ullman and Krasner, 1965). The object was to replace such behaviors with those that were more productive. The distinction is now increasingly blurred between clinical *therapy* and behavioral *influence*, as defined by Ullman and Krasner: "Behavioral influence is the more generic term and includes advertising, brainwashing, institutional pressure, and so forth (as well as psychotherapy) as techniques altering the subject's behavior, whether to increase *adjustive* [italics mine] behavior or not" (1965, p. 1).

Operant conditioning techniques occur in institutions from schoolrooms to zoos. They resonate in a common-sense way with our daily experiences. We *do* work for "rewards." If we can improve the rate

[6] The most elegant critique is provided by Willard Gaylin (1973). See also Eric Fromm's *The Anatomy of Human Destructiveness*, 1973, pp. 34-42, Carl Rogers' response (1956). Shoben (1963), as does Rogers, explores the morality of behavioral modification (clinical sense)—in particular, aversive therapy. Halleck explores the political ramifications (*The Politics of Therapy*, 1971); Arieti (*The Will to Be Human*, 1972, pp. 7-8, 27-29) argues that Skinner prescribes a state *preceding* (his italics) freedom and dignity; see also Chomsky's review (1971). On the matter of creativity, in *The Act of Creation* (1969, p. 157) Arthur Koestler writes:

> Some mechanical virtuosity has probably reached its highest development in the Japanese arts inspired by Zen Buddhism; swordsmanship, archery, judo, calligraphic painting. The method to reach perfection has been authoritatively described as 'practice, repetition, and repetition of the repeated with ever-increasing intensity,' (Herrige) until the adept 'becomes a kind of automaton, so to speak, as far as his own consciousness is concerned' (Suzuki). That is the method by which Professor Skinner of Harvard University, a leader of the Behavioral school, trained pigeons to perform circus acts, intended as an explanation of mental development in man. (p. 157)

Charles Reich, a professor of law at Yale, in *The Greening of America* (1970), a counterculture treatise on the emergence of post-industrial man, doesn't mention Skinner at all.

and size of our "reinforcements," be they love or money, so much the better. It does seem a matter of contingencies and reinforcement. Most of us probably believe that Skinner is, in the long run, more right than wrong. The darker side of behavioral modification is brainwashing, traceable to Pavlov's later experiments (Sargant, 1957), tested in Korea, and more recently in China (Fairbanks, 1973), where effective reinforcement follows starvation. I have also seen certain power and beauty of such techniques. I watched one day a young Oregon teacher using M&M candies as reinforcements to induce the first socializing steps of severely retarded, institutionalized children.

We are equally aware of the power of behavioral modification to accommodate the system, as documented by Goffman (*Asylums*, 1961) and one of Kesey's writings (*One Flew Over the Cuckoo's Nest*, 1962).[7]

Two recent personal discussions bear on the subject. Both pertain to prisons. "Do you think that placing a prisoner in solitary and not telling him how he can get out was cruel and unjust punishment?" asked a lawyer advocate for a Washington State Penitentiary inmate. A second discussion was in conference with a prisoner advocacy law group conconcerned about a behavioral modification treatment program (which also used fluphenazine—Prolixin) in a state prison. My answer to the solitary confinement question was yes, if you were isolated as punishment and provided with no estimate of confinement duration or information as to how you could end the isolation, then this amounted to an instrumental use of anxiety as punishment, and was therefore cruel.

[7] Kanfer (1965) and others—e.g., Crawshaw (1969) on sensitivity training and Edgar (1972) on legal and public policy problems—have also raised questions about the ethics and dangers of such techniques. With reference to positive reinforcement in the public areas, Kanfer stated it as follows:

> Large-scale use of these methods, however, has not concerned people because the age-old deceptions of the Pied Piper have been assumed to be sufficiently transparent to allow most adults to recognize them as false promises and to resist temptation by persuasion. Recently, Browning's Pied Piper of Hamlin has become more sophisticated. He has put on the disguise of a grey flannel suit, of a human relations expert, a psychotherapist, or a friendly interrogator in a prison camp. His pipe has turned into other instruments promising such sweet things as affection and happiness to a juvenile delinquent, money back guaranteed satisfaction with soaps and cereals, or a political paradise for all the masses, all without pain, coercion, or physical violence. This increased professionalism and sophistication in the application of psychologic principles has caused uneasiness to the public because the methods have lost some of their transparency . . . (p. 190)

The behavioral modification experiment truned out not to be experimental. Its level of funding and staffing were not commensurate with its goals; pharmacologic inactivation with drugs was high enough to produce not only a "Prolixin shuffle" but probable interference with reinforcement itself. I was in agreement with the lawyers and prisoners that it was a coercive response to deal with dissidents, masquerading as a treatment program.

Other Brain Control Technologies

Other brain control technologies have been discussed by Pines (1973) and Ferguson (1973). They include biofeedback, *psi* phenomenon, the status of cyborgs,[8] advancements in the "DITWS" (Dilantin in the water supply) idea, cloning, and genetic engineering schemes outlining ways in which the number of cerebral neurons might be doubled. Such esoterica are interesting but are hardly a match in scale or impact for the enforced brain-growth limitations occurring now in underdeveloped countries. Apropos of the Social Predestination Room of Huxley's Brave New World, where a decanted embryo's brain growth is set by exposure time to an oxygenator, we accomplish the same end simply by providing a low-protein, high-carbohydrate diet (e.g., pop and potato chips in Harlem) to pregnant women. This insures development of fetal cerebral cortices of reduced intellectual capacity. Such a catastrophic low-protein regime nourishes embryo brain growth in possibly half of the pregnant women in the world today. There will be no *alphas* among them. By an extraordinary alteration in diet and sensory enrichment in the first year of life, low numbers of *betas* may be salvageable.

In concluding an overview of brain control methods, we might consider the problem from another angle: How are children politically socialized—that is, how is acceptance and identity with a state conditioned? In this regard we examine questions dealing with political and antireligious training of Soviet children, and also the consequences of child-rearing in a kibbutz.

To combat religion in the U.S.S.R. (Cullen, 1974), antireligion training begins in grade 1, the preeminence of science is upheld, and public rituals, art, and physical and cultural opportunities are

[8] Cyborg from "cybernetic organism": ultimates in man-machine combinations ostensibly designed to supplement self-regulatory functions in order to extend a human's ability to cope with new or alien environments as outer space. For an up-to-date fictional account of the status of cyborgs, Joe Poyer's *North Cape* is recommended. Demand pacemakers and the general new field of *neuroprosthetics* are pertinent clinical directions.

provided children to offset the mysteries and art of the church. Mysticism in all forms is systematically criticized, and teaching emphasizes the rationality of man based on science and social principles. Soviet theorists are not interested in mechanical, but *conscious* control of behavior—identity with the purpose and goals of the state are the goals of citizenship.

Political socialization of Russian children is begun after school starts.[9] (Clawson, 1973) Preschool efforts are confined to the work ethic and the authoritarianism of the family. Because of the traditional Soviet bias against certain types of behavioral research, the high cost of day-care centers, and a curious (and unexplained) disinterest in early child-rearing by "virtually everyone who has ever held top political power in the USSR" (Clawson, p. 711), the family continues to be the early center of authoritarian training. The state holds the parents responsible for the behavior of their children.

Clawson is not entirely convinced of the impact of official dogmatism on the child's behavior, and concludes that "the total profile of Soviet political behavior for the present generation, to the extent that it is rooted in early childhood socialization, is more likely to be influenced by the indirect effects of urbanization than by regime-oriented, deliberate political socialization."

In the United States, we have witnessed the disappearance of the nuclear family and a rise in interest in child-care programs (Goocher, 1969), but most world-wide interest has focused on the consequence of raising children in a communal setting—i.e., the kibbutz.

In Bettelheim's study of communal child-rearing in the Israeli kibbutz (*The Children of the Dream*, 1969), after a comparative review of personality development in the kibbutznik and the American child (Erikson's view, 1950), he makes the comment apropos of the consequences of state rearing:

> The existential despair that seems to haunt Western society the kibbutznik escapes: despair about oneself or the world, about the fact that one's life is to end, and that it had little meaning or purpose. But in terms of all I have said, the kibbutznik escapes at a price. By now it should be clear what that consists of. In terms of Erikson's model, despair is escaped at some cost to personal identity, emotional intimacy, and individual achievement. On the other hand, this may seem a very small price to

[9] Soviet mothers have historically shown little interest in preschool socialization, 'moral education, or patriotic training (Clawson, 1973, p. 79, citing Susan Jacoby, (1971). It was found difficult to keep a preschooler's mind on political business. business.

> many of our aging and aged who suffer a feeling of uselessness, a sharp sense of isolation, because there is nothing meaningful for them to do any more, nor any place of importance in society. (p. 318)

Experiments utilizing various brain control techniques to learn about brain function as well as behavior in animals and man are now world-wide. The results are generally "open to the public," available in scientific libraries to all who can read the specialized literature. If explicit application is demanded by an "iron government," what will be the response of neuroscientists? My third premise is: They will deliver.

DELIVERY

> Science, as long as it limits itself to the descriptive study of the laws of nature, has no moral or ethical quality, and this applies to the physical as well as the biologic sciences.
>
> Sir Ernst Chain (cf. Rose and Rose, 1973)

> "We send them up, who cares where they come down. That's not my department," says Werner von Braun.
>
> Tom Lehrer (A song from the 1950's)

> [On scientific knowing] It seeks a neutral eye, an impersonal eye . . . in effect, the eyes of the dead wherein reality is reflected without emotional distortion.
>
> Theodore Roszak, *Where the Wasteland Ends* (1973)

Iron governments will demand adherence to rules, a benevolent synchrony of effort to help people survive hard times. Brain controls will be used for three reasons: first, to adjust individual behavior to the System; second, as treatments to help people "cope" with their crises; and lastly, new techniques will enable more of the ill, the criminal, and the dissident to return to the System. Where this proves impossible, such individuals will be sheltered and isolated if necessary. The need for brain control techniques by an iron government is clear. But how will the link between information and application be provided? This brings us to our third premise having to do with scientists, neuroscientists in particular.

The scientist and technologist will come to power in the decades ahead. The road to success will be education, specialization, and meritocracy.[10] Scientists will be asked to serve the government. When called upon, they will "deliver" brain control technology to the state, resolving what conflicts they have possibly with drugs of their own invention.

Delivery will not be seen as such. It will be walled off from consciousness by processes inherent to science. In the usual sane and detached manner, indistinguishable from that found in work on lunar crystals, cerebellar neurons, or cyclic AMP, methods of brain control will be described, tested, and critically reviewed. In an indifferent but careful manner—dicta of rigorous science—such information will be forwarded painlessly to the state. That is the charge. What is the evidence?

Several aspects of science today bear on the thesis of "delivery." They include the selection of training of scientists; systems of recognition and reward; and the facts that most scientists are economically dependent upon public funds and emotionally dependent upon collective myths which add to their vulnerability on the "delivery" issue.

Esoteric research requires preoccupation and intense concentration, a "tamped-down" view, and detachment from the world around the laboratory. In a science of reductionism with its excitement of discovery of molecular mechanisms, one knows well one small piece of the world at the expense of being provincial and safely unconcerned about the potentially adverse consequences of one's work. It is the rare person that can see beyond the first-order effects of his own efforts. Scientists are no exception. As specialization in the sciences increases, it becomes necessary to accept the expertise or control of others for things beyond one's own knowledge or experience: this is the essence of an interdependent society. As scientists achieve a superfunction status in a future state, the privacy of alienation itself may be

[10] Daniel Bell (*The Coming of Post-Industrial Society*, 1973) adopts this view of the development of a powerful scientific and technologic elite crucial to the operation of a complex technocracy. A similar hope was expressed in *New Atlantis*, Sir Francis Bacon's utopian novel published two centuries ago. For a "class" action critique of Bell's position, especially the central role of ideal science and not-so-ideal normal scientists, see Michael Marien's essay (1973) "Daniel Bell and the End of Normal Science." This source is particularly useful as it provides a history of the term "post-industrial age" (not unique to Bell) and also an extensive bibliography, which could admirably serve as a data base for Heilbronner's essay discussed at the beginning of this paper.

their principal reward. At this point, we note, scientific work and "delivery" would become one and the same.

What are myths of science that make scientists amenable to control and "delivery"? We shall not dwell on the economic dependency of scientific work on state funds. As things now stand, the peer review and grant award system provides a buffer between what a scientist does and what a state might need. But there are indications that this arrangement between the state and scientists will change. The state will undoubtedly set the priorities in the future.

The myths are those that bear on the question of the responsibilities of science to a nonscientist public. Such myths have been explored by many in an attempt to understand the failure of technocracy to fulfill the spiritual needs of men, to celebrate and not destroy individual uniqueness.

Stephen and Hillary Rose (1973) have isolated three myths which focus on responsibility; the idea that the scientific method or Science per se is neutral; the notion of a technologic imperative that translates *can* implies *ought*; and the assertion that scientific findings of importance are accidental, an argument in favor of a science independent of man. Neutral science is the idea of a working scientist who makes no choices; if choices are made, the values are explicit; the values which are applied are universal; and so forth to a vanishing point. That *can* implies *ought* is the technocratic pressure to accomplish and to achieve without regard to cost or consequence. As so often happens, judgment follows accomplishment, and resources and lives may be lost in passage. The idea of an accidental science—the serendipitous observation, the great discovery made while at a tavern (I know of one such case) or somewhere other than a laboratory—is a wonderful myth, a belief that honors the power and beauty of science as being above and apart from human activity.

Myths as these pervade the selection and training of scientists. Interest lies in the selection of intelligence, "proven performance" (good grades), and basic skills. Nonessential skills, an irregular academic performance (the reasons unimportant), or any indications from the applicant of uncertainty about his life or purpose are disqualifying marks. The training of graduate students is not for creativity or an iconoclastic view, the individual who will "bring down the house" (every graduate student's dream); instead, it is aimed at training individuals to perform what Kuhn (1962) called "normal" science, a science of small, careful, logical steps—like accretions to a coral reef—without making mistakes, gambling, or taking big chances. Such "normal" science is beautifully designed to accept and reinforce certain cognitive needs that appear part of the self-selection process of getting into Science and staying there. Maslow (1966), in exploring the roots of a mechanistic, normal science, saw the following cognitive characteristics as useful to the "normal" scientist: a compulsive need to be certain, a denial of doubt or confusion, inflexibility, the need to appear strong and powerful, intolerance or contempt for ambiguity, the need to conform, and more importantly, an overrespect for authority.

Programs of scientific training are anchored to such motifs as "normal science," and reinforcements of such cognitive needs requisite to professional survival. This being so, training itself walls off from consciousness, fears of doubt, ambiguity, and confusion, doing little to strengthen a scientist's identity or responsibility to his human community. He becomes instead a member of the science community.

The myth of neutral science simply means that in the laboratory you're not your brother's keeper. What is found out with patience, good sense, and technical skill are universal things verifiable about nature. If it's a new compound which cures leukemia, we're in luck; if it leads instead—after a long latent period—to development of leukemia, that's bad luck, but then we've learned something new. And so it goes. It is the Launch Philosophy all over again: "We send them up, who cares where they come down? That's not my department, etc." An ability to be nonrational, noncontrolling, and noninterfering is not selected for in today's scientist. This may be his undoing.

Roszak explores this dilemma of scientists in his penetrating critique, *Where the Wasteland Ends*, arguing that in the "citadel of expertise" a puritanical adherence to the objective quest binds the scientist to the state. It thus becomes impossible for the individual scientist to see himself or his work in the wider context of a surrounding world.

This same idea, expressed in various ways, can be found in the writings of Galbraith, Marcuse, Reich, Fromm, and others puzzling over how it is that the brilliant promise of the Industrial Age and its electronic technocracy has not only failed to serve man, but has destroyed his sense of community and provided the work alienation and isolation felt by so many today.

The Methods Problem

One of the intriguing questions about the "delivery" premise is centered in the day-to-day operations of a career. It concerns publishing. To do scientific work and not to publish is absurd. It is professional suicide for those without academic sinecure. Not to "deliver," as the word is used here, is not to publish, and not to publish concludes a scientific career. But it is not publishing per se that is important to the premise of "delivery." All scientists are obliged to publish and thereby enhance public knowledge in all areas of human interest. The problem lies in the format of the scientific paper itself. I speak here of the section called *Methods*. Providing *Methods* to colleagues in the scientific world at large is the *sine qua non* of work. Without a *Methods* section, all would agree that the work is unpublishable. It makes a critical evaluation of the data presented impossible. But it is adherence to this rule alone which makes it absolutely impossible for a scientist to exercise control over the consequences of his contribution. It is *the* Achilles heel, the rule of "delivery" itself, the guarantee that brain control or for that matter any piece of scientific work will automatically be passed to the state.

Scientists have social concerns and have taken unpopular views which at times have jeopardized their careers. Some examples are refusal to work on military projects, heading up public groups to battle vested corporate or political interests—e.g., environmental pollution, denunciation of experiments such as that which occurred at Tuskegee, and more recently the heated debates over psychosurgery. Groups of scientists have formed to discuss the broader issues of ethics and social responsibility—e.g., The Hastings Center Institute of Society, Ethics, and Life Sciences; British Society for Social Responsibility in Science. In the past, where activities of the technocracy or the science itself were directly threatening to man,[11] or we were heading in the direction of a "dystopia"—Sibley's (1973) lovely word for ideal, evil-type states[12]—scientists or the state might call a halt to what was going

[11] For a sobering lesson in the linking of a scientific advancement and its eventual application in war as well as the Berkeley campus riots—the development of the control gas CS—see Rose and Rose (1973) "Can science be neutral?" pp. 610-616.

[12] Huxley's *Brave New World* and *Brave New World Revisited* (1965), Orwell's *1984* (1949), Kurt Vonnegut, Jr.'s *Player Piano* (1967), and more specific dystopic consequences of a technology that lead to nuclear war, as Nevil Shute's *On the Beach* (1957), Roshwald's *Level Seven* (1959), and Miller's *A Canticle for Leibowitz* (1959). I am indebted to M.W. Sibley's paper "Utopian thought and technology" (1973); it provided perspective in the transition of the American state toward another age, a historical context beginning with the Book of Genesis.

on. The options are to either reject technologic advancement[13] (the SST decision can be cited as an example), or to be selective in what is accepted.[14]

These things having been said, the fact remains, however, that by training, dogma, profession, and belief, scientists of the future, in their rise to more powerful positions of influence, will be then, as now, mandated to not interfere with or comprehend the long-term possibilities of their work. They will deliver. At this time there are no other practical options.

DOUBLE AGENTS

> When an individual seeks help from a psychiatrist, he must usually reveal a great deal of embarrassing and potentially condemnatory information about himself. The patient has no alternative since almost all psychiatric techniques are ineffective unless he is willing to reveal himself honestly. Sometimes his honesty costs him dearly; information shared with the psychiatrist can be used to deny the patient important privileges and to deprive him of the ability to influence those around him.
>
> Seymour Halleck, *The Politics of Therapy* (1971)

[13] In *Islandia* (1942, 1958), August Tappen Wright's monumental utopian novel, the citizens decided to reject the advance of technology into their country. Islandians were not convinced that change was good in and of itself. What were the social and psychological consequences? Lord Dorn, at the council on the question of "opening" the country (to technologic instruments):

> 'The way of life of the foreigner has changed completely in the last few hundred years, and changes daily at what seems an accelerating rate. Who dares tell us that a thing so new and so unfixed is good for us? . . . They move too fast to see more than the surface glitter of a life too swift to be real . . . The rush of life past them they call progress, though it is too rapid for them to move with it." (*Islandia*, p. 496)

In *The New Industrial State* Galbraith reviews the response of the industrial system to a community that rejects the system (see chapter 30; the same theme in eloquent detail is found in the third of Goodwin's articles in the *New Yorker*, "The American condition—III," February 4, 1973).

Zeo Prizner, a Marxian radical and boat builder currently constructing a geodesic dome house on Waldron Island in the San Juans, told me that the islanders have recently rejected the notion of a central power and refused county police protection, as well as marinas and improvements in roads, wanting little of technology and new advancements (except domes!).

[14] Aldous Huxley's *Island* (New York: Harper & Row, 1962). The defender of the old ways (Pala): "Electricity plus heavy industry minus birth control equals democracy and plenty. Electricity, plus heavy industry minus birth control equals misery, totalitarianism, and war" (cited by Sibley, 1973 p. 275). This selective utopia eventually gave way to technologic and development pressures.

> After all, the question is not whether Sakharov enjoys intellectual freedom: there is no doubt that he does. The question is how he uses it and for what purpose.
>
> M.V. Keldysh, President of the Soviet Academy of Science

With the rise of an iron government, availability of new brain control techniques and "delivery" by neuroscientists, we come to two sticky questions: who will the state get to administer the controls? And, as Kenneth Clark was asked,[15] Who controls the controllers?

Unhappily, the first job will fall to physicians—in particular, psychiatrists—as I shall try to show. The matter of who controls the controllers in the iron government envisioned earlier is a more difficult question—given the assumption that the kind of iron government we are talking about will be a pluralism of bureaucracies and planning, whirring away like a giant clock, a total bureaucracy of people-functions. In such a vague model, it is the logic and arrangements of equilibrium points within such a planned society that provide the control of the controller: the controller of the controller is not unlike the controller of social amenities between people as they meet for the first time. The controls are evident, as greeting behavior is stereotyped, but there is no identifiable or written controller. Saying this, we turn next to focus specifically on the psychiatrist as the probable agent of the state on the use of brain controls.

It is unlikely that there is a physician in this country today who would not disavow a willingness to be used as a puppet by the state—in the context of the brain control issue—to knowingly suppress dissent, administer punishment to prisoners, or "warehouse" mental patients as a substitute for treatment. In exploring this executioner question, it is not my intent to malign psychiatry as I pursue in a speculative manner the dark question: who will be the bagman for brain control in the future? It is at worst a dreadful

[15]In Kenneth Clark's Presidential Speech to the American Psychological Association on September 4, 1971, he suggested that a drug be developed that would be administered to those in power to prevent them from using power unwisely. The call for a *peace pill* provoked a violent protest from colleagues, politicians, and the public. Clark felt that the public reaction was indicative of a threat to the idea of the omniscience of leaders and their presumed normal mental and moral health. To the question—who controls the controllers—Clark simply responded: who controls the people that now control? Clark concluded that most people didn't care as long as it *wasn't* a psychologist (Warren, 1973).

aspersion. At best, it may help to continue a consciousness-raising about such questions (Chodoff, 1974).

It should be noted at the outset that casting the psychiatrist in this fearful role is not new. It is a conclusion of those outside psychiatry exploring the sociology of institutions (Goffman, 1961), investigating how women may be treated if they abandon male-defined roles (Chesler, 1972), or attempting to demonstrate the class structure of mental illness (Hollingshead and Redlich, 1958). The same suggestion can also be found in the psychiatric literature—e.g., Szasz (*Myth of Mental Illness,* 1961), Halleck (*The Politics of Therapy,* 1971), Menninger (*The Crime of Punishment,* 1968), and Laing (*The Politics of Experience and the Bird of Paradise,* 1971). Historical antecedents are given in papers tracking the role of psychiatrists in commitment proceedings (Szasz, 1973). And more recently it can be found in studies of bureaucratic attitudes in mental hospitals (Ottenberg, 1974), and in the concerns of a generation of new psychiatry residents who suspect the worst (Mandell, 1973).

The question of the psychiatrists future role on brain control vis-à-vis the state can be divided into two parts: a section on drugs and a section on the *double agent* problem. Before reviewing the drug question, we must first dispense with the implausible idea that psychiatrists would ever accept or perform as brain control agents for the state.

Taken at face value, the premise that psychiatrists will be the agent and provide the legitimacy for brain control techniques for the future state is absurd. Most psychiatrists are independently employed and do not work for the state. While they may use their therapeutic role to adjust a patient's life to better accept his fate, they remain free agents in a fee-for-service system with the autonomy they need to use their best judgment for each patient. Further, there is little evidence that psychiatrists have participated or are interested in legislative or political matters (Suarez, 1972), or that their involvement in politics makes much of an impression (Jus, 1973). Their group efforts to deal with such difficult questions as dyssocial behavior or violence are not impressive (Miller and Auerbach, 1973). Psychiatrists who do pursue more sociotherapeutic careers and locate in culture "hot spots" have a short professional half-life (Bolman, 1972), as do their ideas (Arthur, 1972; Glasscote, 1971). And their impact on the criminal law system has been not only meager but subservient, as suggested by Suarez (1972):

> Psychiatry has been involved with the criminal law system for quite some time. But to date this has not been a happy, or for that matter, a productive relationship. The history of collaboration between these two

> disciplines reveals that psychiatry has typically become involved at the request of the legal process, and worse, that the tasks and roles to be performed have been delineated and defined by the legal system rather than by psychiatry. (p. 69)

Thus, by virtue of a private practice life, essential noninvolvement or noneffective involvement in the social, legislative, and political life of the country (with some notable exceptions—e.g., Robert Coles), how is it that the psychiatrist is seen as playing a crucial role in an emerging totalitarian society?

Drugs

Psychiatrists are the most knowledgeable professionals we have in the use of psychotropic drugs. They are licensed to use them to treat patients who in their clinical judgment will benefit from their use. I shall assume that this license and knowledge will continue. Three aspects of drug use are of interest. The first has to do with drug use for mental illness. What do we do if the number of drugs expand so that all behavior can be altered to better harmonize with state needs? Let us, for example, define Halloween mischief as an age-dependent dyssocial act; those above a certain age are viewed not as pranksters but as persons who have committed a dyssocial act. Given a new drug that will suppress such acts, are we not defining the act as mental illness? If we aren't, then the drug is given to control dyssocial behavior. Klerman (1972) has considered this same question:

> As the population becomes more confident in the technologic capacity of psychiatrists and other mental health professionals, there is a broadening in the definition of mental illness. Larger segments of the population are now seeking help from mental health professions for problems which were not defined previously as "illnesses." The pace has accelerated so much that much of social deviance, previously regarded as illegal, is in the process of being redefined as mental illness. In this redefinition, there is the hope that the technology that has proved useful for schizophrenia, depression, and related mental illnesses will also prove successful in *altering deviant behavior such as alcoholism and perhaps even crime and delinquency.* [Italics mine]

Klerman suggests that new drugs may bring dyssocial behavior under control, making such behavior—as in the case of the MBD-diagnosed child—a brain disorder by virtue of the doctrine *res ipsa loquitor*.

A second problem is the likelihood that as our century advances, more adults will be on psychotropic agents to cope with their personal lives. In this case, drugs will be prescribed to provide a modicum of comfort or escape. Physicians and psychiatrists will be charged with the duty of monitoring the safe use of such drugs for an increasing number of people. Psychiatrists will have the role of treating an individual's response to cultural crises. The drug indirectly legitimates the idea that it is the individual's weakness and not that of his society. The psychiatrist in this situation needs no external controller. He is acting in the context of healer.

Lastly, there is the use of drugs by the state psychiatrist to subdue or isolate political dissidents or to destroy their creditability of sanity.

In the psychotic individual, ataractic drugs *improve* civil liberty (R. Kimball, personal communication) as they improve the ability to think and argue more effectively. The same drugs given to you or me produce lethargy and withdrawal. Drug use by deceit to destroy a person's intellect or creditability in the service of a state interested in isolating dissidents could be accomplished by producing either an overt (LSD) or more subtle (mescaline) psychomimetic reaction.

Psychiatrists as Double Agents

The concept of a double agent is the idea of a person serving two masters. In the United States, the double agent role occurs principally in three institutions—viz., prisons, mental hospitals, and in military services. It has been argued that psychiatrists in these institutions adjust the behavior of their charges to the norms or convenience of the institution first, and the needs of the patients to outer society second. This is certainly true of the military (Caldwell, 1967) and prisons (Rundel, 1972); to what extent it occurs in mental hospitals is unknown. In the future, when psychiatrists work for the state, will they not serve the state first? A study of the double agent problem in the United States has been promised, but is not yet underway. Its importance lies in answering the question, Given a more totalitarian state, what can be expected of psychiatry?

A fruitful place to begin is with the analysis of the double agent role of the Russian psychiatrist. He is employed by a totalitarian state; one task is to identify and treat political dissent as mental illness. Examination of some recent events in Russia are presented in detail to clarify this point and to underscore its seriousness for psychiatrists everywhere. If exported or applicable here, it supports the premise that in the emergence of an iron government, it falls to psychiatry to direct and administer use of brain control techniques.

In early 1971, Vladimir Bukovsky, a Russian civil rights activist, reported to Western psychiatrists (the "Bukovsky papers"; cf. Chodoff, 1974) that political dissidents in the Soviet Union were being confined to mental institutions. The charge was substantiated in the same year by Zhores Medvedev's published account *A Question of Madness*

(1971) of his similar treatment at Kaluga in the spring of 1970. Medvedev's diagnosis was referred to as the Leonardo da Vinci[16] syndrome; hospitalization was initiated probably because of his anti-Lysenko and civil liberty writings published in the West.[17]

The charges were debated at the World Psychiatry Association Congress in Mexico City in December 1971 and denounced as a cold war plot by A.V. Shnezhnevsky, chief psychiatrist of the U.S.S.R. The Congress took no official action, but the Board of Trustees of the American Psychiatric Association (APA), on December 9, 1971, went on record with a statement "opposing the misuse of psychiatric facilities for the detention of persons solely on the basis of their political dissent, no matter where it occurs."

The charge was that Russian psychiatrists worked as double agents; that, in fact, anyone who politically dissented or embarrassed the state was viewed as mentally ill, recalling the old police-at-the-elbow definition of insanity—if you committed a crime with a policeman at your elbow, you were obviously crazy.

As Rosenham (1973)[18] asked in his now-famous experiment on mental institutions: "If sanity and insanity exist, how shall we know them?"

The APA set up an Ad Hoc Committee on Use of Psychiatric Institutions for the Commitment of Political Dissenters, which included among its distinguished panel the respected jurist David Bazelon (Durham decision), Chief Justice of the Court of Appeals, Washington, D.C. The group decided the Bukovsky papers were authentic, directed the APA trustees to circulate the APA's position statement internationally, and also recommended that a commission be appointed to formulate international regulations. A resolution to

[16] The Leonardo da Vinci syndrome is a facetious reference to a widened definition of schizophrenia: e.g., work in two disparate fields—in Medvedev's case, biology and sociology (cited in Rose, 1973, p. 299). In Medvedev's case, the actual diagnosis was "incipient schizophrenia"; paranoid delusions of reforming society (Medvedev and Medvedev, 1971, p. 175).

[17] Medvedev, Z. *The Rise and Fall of T.D. Lysenko*, New York, Columbia University Press, 1971. The other unpublished manuscripts confiscated in February 1971 was *Fruitful Meetings Between Scientists of the World.* It and *Secrecy of Correspondence is Guaranteed by Law* was later published in the United States in one volume, *The Medvedev Papers* (New York: Macmillan, 1971).

[18] D.L. Rosenham's study "On being sane in insane places," *Science* 179:250-258, 1973, suggested that it may not be possible, at least by the methods he used, to distinguish the sane from the insane in psychiatric institutions, a finding independent of malice or stupidity.

do this effect was sent to the World Psychiatric Association, which to this date has taken no action.

Bazelon also suggested to the APA that the situation should also be examined in the United States (Ezra Pound and General Edwin Walker's hospitalizations were famous cases in point). To what extent did the double agent problem as well as other deficiencies in institutional psychiatry exist in the United States?

A grant (APA) was provided and a staff chosen to begin work in January 1973 on "conflict of interest" issues as practiced by psychiatrists under institutional employ. By June 1973, the staff had been "dehired," and a squabble broke out over the reasons why (Miller, 1973). Bazelon charged and the APA denied that psychiatrists were unwilling to examine the evidence and consequence of alleged double agent roles (Bazelon, 1973; APA's committee controversy, 1973).

As this controversy continued, a new charge on the same theme threatened the détente developing between the United States and the USSR. In late August 1973, Andrei Sakharov, a Russian theoretical physicist, reiterated Medvedev's charges about Soviet use of psychiatry to punish political activists.[19] These charges eventually led

[19] After the August 21, 1973 press conference to Western reporters, Sakharov [who had opposed détente as long as the U.S.S.R. remained a secret, repressive society (Bengelsdorf, 1973), a position presented in *Thoughts on Progress, Coexistence*, and *Intellectual Freedom*, 1968—unpublished in Russia] was denounced in Pravda by a letter of August 29, 1973, signed by forty Soviet academicians, five of whom were foreign associates of the National Academy of Science (NAS) of the United States. A similar letter attacking Sakharov from the Siberian division of the Soviet Academy appeared on September 3, 1973. Both letters charged that Sakharov had distorted Soviet reality. Philip Handler, president of the NAS, warned the Soviets on September 8, 1973 (text published in *Science* "News and Comment," 1973), that any repressive acts against Sakharov would jeopardize existing U.S.-Soviet scientific exchange programs. M.V. Keldysh (who was thoroughly familiar with the Medvedev case) of the Soviet academy replied on October 17, 1973 (*Science*, "News and Comment," 1973), objected to the fact and tone of Handler's letter, and stated that U.S. comments on the Sakharov case were not accurate: "After all, the question is not whether Sakharov enjoys intellectual freedom; there is no doubt that he does. The question is how he uses it and for what purpose." Handler replied to Keldysh ("Briefing," 1973), thanking him for his assurances, and stated that he was appalled by the terrorist intimidation (that Sakharov had apparently experienced). He was privately pleased that the Soviets were willing to talk about the Sakharov case. A month later, in November 1973, Yuri A. Kjikhanovich, a forty-one-year-old Moscow State University mathematician who had been held incommunicado for fourteen months, was finally examined at Serbski Institute after nine months of imprisonment and pronounced mentally incompetent to stand trial for political activities. Sakharov, an attendant at the hearing, reported that the diagnosis was a slowly developing form of schizophrenia ("Prominent psychiatrists protest . . . " 1973).

to a semiofficial inquiry by an international group of psychiatrists which included the APA president, Dr. Alfred Freedman. A meeting was held at Serbski in November in the Soviet Union. The discussions were widely reported in the psychiatric press ("Soviets agree . . .," 1973; "Freedman . . .," 1973; "Soviets discuss . . .,"1973), but nothing important emerged except for the fact that the Soviet psychiatrists saw things differently than their Western counterparts (as Allen's 1973 comparative study had shown); that they believed in many forms of schizophrenia, and besides, they are saving their patients from the brutalities of Siberian exile, a concession reported of Alexander Volpin—i.e., that being in a psychiatric hospital had probably saved his life (Ottenberg, 1974).

As things now stand, we appreciate more clearly a potential unpleasant role for psychiatrists in the service of a totalitarian state. And more attention is being given to the bureaucratic inertia in mental institutions in this country, which in effect saddle the psychiatrist with a double agent role weighted to the institution (Ottenberg, 1974).

As we approach the end of the century, a transition period predictably stormy, the question of invasion of privacy can also be added to the list of challenges. Invasion of privacy at all levels is now a national issue. Privacy, quoting Kanfer (1965), "the inaccessibility of much personal behavior in a democratic society, probably represents the bulwark of democracy because it allows for variability, and for divergence of attitudes and beliefs. It is also a crucial question for the psychiatrist as what is jealously guarded privacy in everyday life, must be surrendered in the psychotherapeutic interview." How will this arrangement fare in the office of a state-appointed psychiatrist in a future iron government?

In concluding this section on psychiatrist as double agents, how realistic is our premise, given the current private practice model, an open society, and considerable judicial statutes protecting the rights of the individual recommended for commitment? Things change, and we have reason to worry on several scores.

Socialized medicine in the United States is rapidly expanding, and fee-for-service medicine (except for after hours and the "carriage trade") will probably disappear. Psychiatrists, too, will work for the state; their roles perhaps won't change on the surface, but their mission will: reduce the dissonance and stress of people trying to survive in trying times.

A second concern is that psychiatrists will be controlled to neutralize their danger to the state because of their accustomed freedom and hence unpredictableness, especially in situations of social chaos. Halleck's (1971) chilling speculations on how a psychiatrist might serve a ruthless university administrator in putting down a student strike is required reading for those doubtful of the power or likelihood of the double agent promise. His comparison of the difference between a "conservative" and a "radical" psychiatrist's management of a community mental health center additionally suggests that because of their unpredictableness and different training, state control of the psychiatrists will be necessary.

Other reasons include the state's probable takeover of the now all but financially bankrupt American medical school system, gaining here the ability to select and train physicians for a role in a quite different and totally planned society, in which the individual-as-function will be the therapeutic target.

Thus the psychiatrist, as time passes, will come under intense scrutiny. His role as agent for Big Brother will not seem to be that. Big Brother will be no elite group or person, but instead will be a compelling system (iron government) organized to maximize each individual's opportunities as it delineates a citizen's special function in a more crowded, fearful, and interdependent world of limited resources and lessened opportunity. The application of brain controls will be a matter of degree. Hopefully the dictum "that control which is least is best" will prevail. But the short straw goes to the psychiatrist and, to a lesser degree, to all physicians. And, as privately observed by Russian psychiatrists, those upon whom such duties fall shall also be monitored.

OPEN AGENDA

In setting forth premises about how brain controls will emerge and who will use them in a democratic society in transition, let them serve as the grounds for arguments, not despair. In logic, if premises are granted as true, a conclusion (e.g., to a syllogism) necessarily follows. But there can be, in the context of society, many alternative conclusions. How we respond to challenges provides the stage for consequences.

In exploring our changing society and its worries about brain controls, it seemed wisest to focus first on premises having to do with development, need, and use of controls rather than on controls per se. I take as an item of faith that all accept the fact that societies are based on controls, those laws, traffic signs, and coercive rules of social demeanor that are implicit or explicit in everything from child-rearing practices, the schoolroom, and work situations to forums, documents, and rituals that keep our lives sorted out. Such controls are designed to make us more predictable in our behavior toward one another. "Freedom and control," as Willard Gaylin (1973) recently said, "are not a moral polarity in anyone's philosophy." Control per se is therefore not the issue.

Instead, we mean those brain controls which invade an individual's privacy, his mental refuge (the residence of soul to some theologians), in such a way that they deprive him, knowingly or unknowingly, of alternative thoughts or choices, the substance of protest, or of grounds for understanding the source of his pain. Brain control abnormally alters the interface between what sensory receptors pass to the brain and the response. By invading the brain with foreign strategies of coercion, we make it possible or impossible to know our world realistically, or to alter it in ways more accountable to our needs. We can and do change minds now to fit environments, but where the fault lies in reality *there* is where we should be working. Should this not be possible in the future?

Let me again set the premises to logical, but dismal ends. In the chaos created by economic decline, a no-growth or equilibrium economy—given other threats (nuclear and environmental) in the struggle over resources—we face the rise of an iron government, a totalitarian outfit with exceptionally broad controls over each citizen's life. Such a society will employ brain controls of a sophisticated type, delivered by psychiatrists or their analogues, to assure survival (by control) of the individual and the state.

But there are alternative conclusions that can be drawn from the premise of hard times. Can we not deploy the technocracy and its communication network first to accurately assess the dimensions of our predicament, and then to set forth alternatives? Can we not make use of the "liberty machine" idea of Stafford Beer (1972), a computer network scattered over the globe monitoring data on industrial, social, and biologic events to provide on-line information and estimates useful to wise decisions? Could not such centers be interconnected to produce—in Michael Arbib's (1973) language—a man-machine symbiosis, the use of technology to solve our difficulties, including those of a legal nature; a balancing of the rights of individuals against the technocratic state, a theory of justice (Rawls, 1971) commensurate to changing times? In asking that we use our technocracy to redesign and restore our community, we do so not only with computers in mind, but also with architects, lawyers, poets and play-rights, and the multitude of talented persons at hand in need of such a community, a place. This faces up to the no-growth crisis.

The question of brain control technology puts the question unfairly. That it is an outgrowth of brain research is true, but that such techniques can serve only dictators is nonsense. Questions of brain control and dyssocial behavior will become more difficult, and there is a potential for great mischief. But the issue can cut both ways: careful use of amphetamines in selected MBD children does improve the life of the child and may save a family; and psychotropic drugs can settle thinking into more self-preserving modes. There is no reason that *enhancement* of intrinsic brain functions, such as memory, insight, planning, judgment, etc., needed to survive and celebrate existence in another era cannot also be explored. Another word than "control" is needed, but it would add much to current work and discussion of civil liberty and privacy questions if we consider the possibility that brain research may lead to techniques to promote more, rather than lessen, brain privacy. Such brain agents or controls might serve transition-period man well.

What scientists will do vis-à-vis the government's request for controls to sedate or robotize a populace is hard to say. But it is conceivable that neuroscientists may opt to draft an oath or code of ethics which states in effect that their studies shall not be designed to provide the means for or assist in the capture of the executive faculties of thought of another human being, where such capture is knowingly detrimental to an individual's liberty or as a coercion for State purposes. The selection, training, and work of a scientist as a function of community and not of science-at-large could also be explored, not to the detriment of science but for its enhancement as service.

In suggesting the future psychiatrist as the likely *double agent* between individuals and the state, we have unfairly assumed it to go only one way—viz., the psychiatrist will use available technology to tune a dysfunctional individual to state needs. But future psychiatrists could be viewed as ombudsman, and if legally granted autonomy from the state (as I think absolutely necessary), then it is possible to see the double agent role in a very different light.

In an iron government of the future, I want my psychiatrist to be a Renaissance individual, a spokesman to adjust not me, but my state, or at least to negotiate between us. As a "free" double agent, the psychiatrist of the future should be empowered to adjust or have adjusted either the state or me to bring us into harmony. What's good for the goose (tranquilizers) is good for the gander (a new IC chip or subroutines in the community computer). In this way, brain controls themselves become an "open agenda."

In closing, these many issues require a deep and wide discussion throughout the country, from classrooms to art studios, from legislative chambers to the space around laboratory coffeepots and blackboards, and across dinner tables everywhere.

As we approach our two hundredth birthday as a nation, brain control should be an "open agenda"—a public issue, informed, argumentative, with all being heard. Our institution of democracy now depends upon it. It will not be easy, but as Max said, in my son Peter's favorite book—*Where the Wild Things Are* (Sendak, 1963)—"let the wild rumpus start."

ACKNOWLEDGMENTS

A number of people read and discussed the manuscript in its early draft, bringing to it a wealth of insight, concern, and criticism that was gratefully appreciated. Discussions with Hal and Crista Markowitz and my wife, Nancy, explored sources of discontent and alienation within the context of a Skinnerian world and what options we have. Curt Boylls, Lee Robertson, and Curtis Bell made substantial changes in the major premises to make them more clear. Lew Nashner and Curt Boylls provided a penetrating critique of contemporary science and its educational directives, and Lew introduced me to Maslow's writings. Sharon Spray reminded me about the problem of women and madness. Bill and Sue Roberts pointed out that controls are intrinsic to democratic institutions, that drugs in children can save families, and that there are positive features to more socialized, less wealthy societies (Sweden). Howard Dewey noted that we cannot afford our alienation between science and community much longer. Will Larson gave assurances that the best of medicine would prevail in the future and added his usual grace of language. Barbara and Reid Kimball sharpened the psychiatric and drug issues on the matter of the ill and non-ill; and Ralph Crawshaw shared with me his recent visit to Russia and the double agent question of Soviet psychiatrists.

M.C. Donner typed and edited the manuscript with the care to which I've become accustomed; and residents and colleagues alike in the Institute permitted my month's retreat without complaint; such time was subtracted from my work on Grant No. NB02289-15 (N.I.H.).

REFERENCES

Allen, M.G. Psychiatry in the United States and the USSR: A comparison. *Amer. J. Psychiat.* 130:1333-1337, 1973.

Andy, O.J., and Jurko, M.F. Thalamotomy for hyperresponsive syndrome. In *Psychosurgery*, E. Hitchcock, L. Laitinen, and K. Vaernet (eds.). Springfield, Illinois: Charles C Thomas, 1972, p. 127-135.

"APA's committee controversy—A rebuttal." *Psychiatric News*, November 21, 1973.

Arbib, M.A. Man-machine symbiosis and the evolution of human freedom. *American Scholar* 43:38-54, 1973-74 edition.

Ardrey, R. *The Territorial Imperative.* New York: Atheneum, 1966.

Arieti, S. *The Will to Be Human.* New York: Quadrangle Books, 1972.

Arthur, R.J. Prevention of "future shock." *New Engl. J. Med.* 237:311-312, 1972.

Avis, H. The neuropharmacology of aggression: a critical review. *Psych. Bull.* 81:47-63, 1973.

Azrin, N.H. Punishment of elicited aggression. *J. Exp. Annals Behav.* 14:7-10, 1970.

Bach y Rita, G., Lion, J.R., Climent, C.E., and Ervin, F.R. Episodic dyscontrol: A study of 130 violent patients. *Amer. J. Psychiat.* 127:1473-1478, 1971.

"Bazelon says psychiatry resists self-scrutiny." *Psychiatric News*, August 8, 1973.

Beer, S. The liberty machine. In *Cybernetics, Artificial Intelligence, and Ecology*, H.W. Robinson and D.E. Knight (eds.). New York: Spartan Books, 1972.

Bell, D. *The Coming of Post-Industrial Society: A Venture in Social Forecasting.* New York: Basic Books, 1973.

Bengelsdorf, I.S. Letter to Pravda. *Science* 182:334, 1973.

Bettelheim, B. *The Children of the Dream.* Toronto: Macmillan, 1969.

Birnbaum, M. The right to treatment. *Amer. Bar. Assoc. J.* 46:499-505, 1960.

Bolman, W.M. Community control of the community mental health center, I: Introduction. *Amer. J. Psychiat.* 129:173-180, 1972.

Breggin, P. The return of lobotomy and psychosurgery. *Congressional Record* 118: E1602-E1612, 1972a.

Breggin, P. Psychosurgery for the control of violence—including a critical examination of the work of Vernon Mark and Frank Ervin. *Congressional Record* 118: E3350-E3386, 1972b.

"Briefing." *Science* 182:371, 1973.

British Society for Social Responsibility in Science. *Manifesto*. London, British Society for Social Responsibility in Science, 1969.

Burke, R.E., Dubner, R., Frank, K., and Hodos, W. "Draft position on psychosurgery." *Neuroscience Newsletter* 4:7, 1973.

Buss, A.H. *The Psychology of Aggression*. New York: Wiley, 1961.

Caldwell, J.M. Military psychiatry. In *Comprehensive Textbook of Psychiatry*, A.M. Freedman and H.I. Kaplan (eds.), Baltimore: William and Wilkins, pp. 1605-1612, 1967.

Chesler, P. *Women and Madness*. New York: Doubleday, 1972.

Chomsky, N. "The case against B.F. Skinner." *The New York Review of Books*, December 30, 1971.

Chodoff, P. Involuntary hospitalization of political dissenters in the Soviet Union. *Psychiatric Opinion*, 11:5-19, 1974.

Clawson, R.W. Political socialization of children in the U.S.S.R. *Pol. Sci. Quart.* 88:684-712, 1973.

Clemente, C.D., and Chase, M.H. Neurologic substrates of aggressive behavior. *Ann. Rev. Physiol.* 35:329-356, 1973.

Clements, S.D. National Project on Minimal Brain Dysfunction in Children—Terminology and Identification, Monograph Number 3. Public Health Service Publication No. 1415, Superintendent of Documents, Government Printing Office, Washington, D.C., 1966.

Crawshaw, R. Community mental health and psychological pollution. *Bull. Menninger Clin.* 35:407-415, 1971.

Crawshaw, R. How sensitive is sensitivity training? *Amer. J. Psychiat.* 126:868-873, 1969.

Crichton, M. *The Terminal Man*. New York: Knopf, 1972.

Cullen, J.B. On the methods, rational and unanticipated consequences of Soviet atheistic "upbringing." *Relig. Educ.* 69:72-87, 1974.

Declaration of Helsinki: Issued by the World Health Association. In *Ann. Int. Med. Suppl.* 7:74-75, 1964.

Dow, R.S., Grimm, R.J., and Rushmer, D.S. Psychosurgery and brain stimulation: the legislative experience in Oregon in 1973. In *Cerebellum, Epilepsy, and Behavior*, I.S. Cooper and M. Riklan, (eds.), New York: Plenum, 1974.

Edgar, H. Legal and public policy problems with behavioral control therapies. A.A.A.S., 139th meeting, New York, December 12, 1972.

Erikson, E.H. *Childhood and Society*. New York: W.W. Norton, 1950.

Fairbanks, J.K. "In Chinese Prisons." *New York Review of Books*, November 1, 1973. (Reviewing *Prisoners of Mao*, Bao Ruo-wang (Jean Pasqualini) and Rudolph Chelminski, London: Coward, McCann and Geoghegan; *China Behind the Mask*, by Warren Phillips and Robert Keatley, New York: Dow-Jones Books; and *A Chinese View of China* by John Fairbanks, New York: Pantheon.)

Federal involvement in the use of behavior modifying drugs on grammar school children. Hearing before a subcommittee of the Committee on Government Operations, House of Representatives, 91st Congress, 2nd session, September 29, 1970, Washington, D.C.: U.S. Government Printing Office, 1970.

Ferguson, M. *The Brain Revolution*. New York: Taplinger, 1973.

Fox, S.S., Copland, R., and Fox, J.J. The new psychiatric prison. Submitted to the National Convention of the National Lawyer's Guild; Austin, Texas, February 1973.

"Freedman reports visit with Soviet psychiatrists." *Psychiatric News*, November 21, 1973.

Freeman, W. Psychosurgery. In *American Handbook of Psychiatry*, Vol. II., pp. 1521-1540, 1959.

Fromm, E. *The Anatomy of Human Destructiveness*. New York: Holt, Rinehart, and Winston, 1973.

Galbraith, J.K. *The New Industrial State*. New York: New American Library, 1968.

Gaylin, W. "Skinner Redux." *Harper's*, October 1, 1973.

Glasscote, R.M. The mental health center: portents and prospects. *Amer. J. Psychiat*. 127:940-941, 1971.

Goffman, E. *Asylums*. Garden City, N.Y.: Anchor Books, 1961, p. 386.

Goldstein, M. Current status for brain research and violent behavior *Arch. Neurol*. 30:1-34, 1974.

Goocher, B.E. "Child Care in the 21st Century." Paper presented at the 2nd annual meeting of the Child Welfare Association of Oregon, Portland, Oregon, April 1969.

Goodwin, R.N. "Reflections: The American Condition." *The New Yorker*, (I) January 21, 1973; (II) January 28, 1974; (III) February 4, 1974.

Grimm, R.J. Advocacy of psychosurgery and intracranial brain stimulation in the involuntarily committed: medical, legal, and ethical objections. Statement of ACLU of Oregon, Senate Human Resources Committee Hearing on SB-298, Oregon Legislature, Salem, Oregon, March 20, 1973.

Grinspoon, L., and Singer, S.B. Amphetamines in the treatment of hyperkinetic children. *Harvard Educational Review* 43:515-555, 1973.

Halleck, S.L. *The Politics of Therapy*. New York: Science House, Inc., 1971.

Heilbroner, R.L. "The human prospect." *New York Review of Books* 20:21-34, 1974.

Hollingshead, A.B., and Redlich, F.C. *Social Class and Mental Illness. A Community Study*. New York: Wiley, 1958.

Horowitz, M.J. *Psychosocial Function in Epilepsy*. Springfield, Ill.; Charles C Thomas, 1970.

Hunsinger, S. School storm: Drugs for children. *Christian Science Monitor*, Oct. 31, 1970, pp. 1-6.

Huxley, A. *Island*. New York: Harper & Row, 1962.

Huxley, A. *Brave New World* and *Brave New World Revisited*. New York: Harper Colophon Books, 1965.

Jacoby, S. Who raises Russian children? *Saturday Review*, August 21, 1971.

Jus, A. Social systems and the criteria of health as defined by the World Health Organization. *Amer. J. Psychiat.* 130:125-131, 1973.

Kaimowitz, Doe, et al. vs. Department of Mental Health for the State of Michigan et al. Civil Action No. 73-19434-AW, Circuit Court for the County of Wayne, Michigan, July 10, 1973.

Kanfer, F.H. Issues and ethics in behavioral manipulation. *Psychol. Reports.* 16:187-196, 1965.

Keniston, K. *The Uncommitted: Alienated Youth in American Society.* New York: Harcourt, Brace & World, 1965.

Kesey, K. *One Flew Over the Cuckoo's Nest.* New York: Viking, 1962.

Klerman, G.L. "Ethical issues on behavior control by new psychotropic drugs." In A.A.A.S. symposium on the ethical and legal issues on new techniques of behavioral control. Washington, D.C., December 27, 1972.

Knight, G.C. Intractable psychoneuroses in elderly and infirm—treatment in stereotactic tractotomy. *Brit. J. Geriatric Practice* 115:257-266, 1966.

Koestler, A. *The Act of Creation.* New York: Macmillan, 1969.

Kuhn, T.S. *The Structure of Scientific Revolutions.* Chicago: University of Chicago Press, 1962.

Ladd, E.T. Pills for classroom peace. *Saturday Review* 53:66-68, 81-83, November 21, 1970.

Laing, R.D. *The Politics of Experience and the Bird of Paradise.* Hammondsworth, Middlesex: Penguin Books Ltd., 1967.

Laitinen, L.V., and Vilkki, J. Stereotaxic ventral anterior cingulotomy in some psychological disorders. In *Psychosurgery,* E. Hitchcock, L. Laitinen, and K. Vaernet (eds.). Springfield, Illinois: Charles C Thomas, 1972, pp. 242-252.

Lansdell, H. "Psychosurgery: some ethical considerations." Talk given at the Council for International Organizations of Medical Sciences (IOMS) on "Protection of Human Rights in the Light of Scientific and Technologic Progress in Biology and Medicine," Geneva, Switzerland, 1973, pp. 14-16.

Leonard, H.L., Epstein, L.J., Bernstein, P., and Ransom, D.C. Hazards implicit in prescribing psychoactive drugs. *Science* 169:438-441, 1970.

Lorenz, K. *On Aggression.* New York: Harcourt Brace Jovanovich, 1966.

Mandell, A.J. Western humanism, modern liberal politics, and psychiatric training: friends or foes? *Amer. J. Psychiat.* 130:529-531, 1973.

Marcuse, H. *One Dimensional Man.* Boston: Beacon, 1964.

Marien, M. Daniel Bell and the end of normal science. *Futurist* 7:262-269, 1973.

Mark, V.H., Brain surgery in agressive epiliptics. *Hastings Center Report* 3:1-5, 1973.

Mark, V.H., and Ervin, F.R. *Violence and the Brain.* New York: Harper and Row, 1970.

Mark, V.H., Sweet, W.H., and Ervin, F.R. Role of brain disease in riots and urban violence. *JAMA* 201:895, 1967.

Maslow, A. *The Psychology of Science.* New York: Harper and Row, 1966.

McConnel, J.V. "Criminals can be brainwashed—now." *Psychology Today,* April 1970.

McGarry, L.A., and Kaplan, H.A. Overview: current trends in mental health law. *Amer. J. Psychiat.* 130:621-630, 1973.

McLuhan, M., and Foore, P. *The Medium is the Message.* London: Allen Lane, The Penguin Press, 1967.

Meadows, D.H., Meadows, D.L., Randers, J., and Behrens, W.H., III. *The Limits of Growth.* Potomac Association Books, 1972.

Medvedev, Z. *Thoughts on Progressive, Peaceful Coexistence and Intellectual Freedom.* New York: Norton, 1968.

Medvedev, Z. *The Medvedev Papers.* New York: Macmillan, 1971.

Medvedev, Z. *The Rise and Fall of T.D. Lysenko.* New York: Columbia University Press., 1971.

Medvedev, Z., and Medvedev, R. *A Question of Madness.* New York: Knopf, 1971.

Menninger, K. *The Crime of Punishment.* New York: Viking, 1968.

Meyer, G., McElhaney, M., Martin, W., and McGraw, C.P., Stereotactic cingulotomy with results of acute stimulation and serial psychological testing in *Surgical Approaches in Psychiatry,* L.V. Laitinen and K.E. Livingston (eds.), Baltimore: University Park Press, 1973, pp. 39-68.

Miller, J. "APA: Psychiatrists reluctant to analyze themselves." *Science* 181:246-248, 1973.

Miller, M.H., and Auerbach, J. Is psychiatry an effective force? *Amer. J. Psychiat.* 130:761-764, 1973.

Miller, W.M., Jr. *A Canticle for Leibowitz.* New York: Lippincott, 1959.

"News and Comment." *Science* 181:1148, 1973.

Nuremberg Code. U.S. Adjutant General's Department. Trials of war criminals before Nuremberg military tribunals under Control Council Law No. 10, The Medical Case, Vol. 2, 1947, 181-183.

"Omaha Pupils Given Behavior Drugs." *Washington Post,* June 29, 1970, pp. 1-8.

Ottenberg, P. Bureaucratic attitudes as a psychosocial defense. *Psychiatric Opinion* 11:26-35, 1974.

Orwell, G. *1984.* New York: Harcourt Brace, 1949.

Physicians' Desk Reference. New Jersey: Medical Economics, 1974.

Pines, M. *The Brain Changers.* New York: Harcourt Brace Jovanovich, 1973.

Platt, J. "What we must do." *Science* 166:1115-1121, 1969.

Poyer, J. *North Cape.* New York: Pyramid, 1969.

Principles of Medical Ethics (pamphlet), American Medical Association, 1957.

Principles of Medical Ethics with Annotations Especially Applicable to Psychiatry. In *Amer. J. Psychiat.* 130:1059-1064, 1973.

"Prominent psychiatrists protest confinement of Soviet dissident." *Psychiatric News,* December 19, 1973.

Ransom, A.J. Social psychiatry: an overview. *Amer. J. Psychiat.* 130:841-849, 1973.

Rawls, J. *A Theory of Justice.* Cambridge, Mass.: Harvard University Press, 1971.

Reich, C.A. *The Greening of America.* New York: Quadrangle Books, 1970.

Robitscher, J. Courts, state hospitals, and the right to treatment. *Amer. J. Psychiat.* 129:74-80, 1972.

Rodham, H. Children under the law. *Harvard Ed. Rev.* 43:487-514, 1973.

Rodin, E. A neurological appraisal of some episodic behavior disturbances with special emphasis on aggressive outbursts given as AC exhibit 3, March 27, 1973, *Kaimowitz, Doe, et al.,* Civil Action No. 73-19434-AW, Circuit Court for the County of Wayne, Michigan, July 10, 1973.

Roeder, F., Orthner, H., and Muller, D. The stereotaxic treatment of pedophilic homosexuality and other sexual deviations. In *Psychosurgery,* E. Hitchcock, L. Laitinen, and K. Vaernet (eds.), Springfield, Ill.: Charles C Thomas, 1972, pp. 87-111.

Rogers, C.R., and Skinner, B.F. "Some issues concerning the control of human behavior: a symposium." *Science* 124:1057-1066, 1956.

Rogers, R.R. Psychiatric hospitalization of political dissenters. *Psychiatric Opinion* 11:20-24, 1974.
Romano-V., O.I. Institutions in modern society: caretakers and subjects. *Science* 183:722-725, 1974.
Rose, S. *The Conscious Brain*. New York: Knopf, 1973.
Rose, S., and Rose, H. Can science be neutral? *Persp. Biol. Med.* 16:605-624, 1973.
Rosenham, D.L. On being sane in insane places. *Science* 179:250-258, 1973.
Roshwald, M. *Level Seven*. London: Heinemann, 1959.
Roszak, T. *The Making of a Counter Culture*. New York: Doubleday, 1969.
Roszak, T. *Where the Wasteland Ends: Politics and Transcendance in Post-Industrial Society*. New York: Doubleday Anchor, 1973.
Rundel, F. The dilemma of a prison doctor. *Hastings Center Report* 2:7-9, 1972.
Safer, D., Allen, R., and Barr, E. Depression of growth in hyperactive children on stimulant drugs. *New England Journal of Medicine*, 287:217-220, 1972.
Sakharov, A.D. *Progress, Coexistence, and Intellectual Freedom*. New York: Norton, 1968.
Sanderson, R., Campbell, D., and Laverty, S. An investigation of a new aversive conditioning technique for alcoholism. In *Condition Techniques in Clinical Practice and Research*, New York: Springer, 1964.
Sargant, W. *Battle for the Mind*. New York: Harper & Row, 1957.
Schneir, W., and Schneir, M. *Invitation to an Inquest*. New York: Doubleday, 1965.
Schwitzgebel, R.K. Development and legal regulations of coercive behavior modification techniques with offenders. NIMH, Public Health Service Publication No. 2067, U.S. Govt. Printing Office, 1971.
Sendak, M. *Where the Wild Things Are*. New York: Harper & Row, 1963.
Shoben, E.J., Jr. The therapeutic object: man or machine? *J. Counsel. Psychol.* 10:264-268, 1963.
Shute, N. *On the Beach*. New York: Morrow, 1957.
Sibley, M.Q. Utopian thought and technology. *Amer. J. Pol. Sci.* 2:255-281, 1973.
Skinner, B.F. *Walden II*. New York: Macmillan, 1962.
Skinner, B.F. *Beyond Freedom and Dignity*. New York: Bantam Books, 1971.
Smith, D.E. Speed freaks versus acid heads: conflict between drug subcultures. *Clin. Peds.* 2:185-192, 1969.
"Soviet Academy replies to NAS defense of Sakharov." *Science* 182:459, 1973.
"Soviets agree to discuss confinement abuses." *Psychiatric News*, October 17, 1973.
"Soviets discuss charges on suppressing dissidents." *Clin. Psychiatric News*, November 1973, p. 4.
Steinfels, P. Confronting the other drug problem. *Hastings Center Report* 2:4-6, 1972.
Suarez, J.M. Psychiatry and the criminal law system. *Amer. J. Psychiat.* 129:69-73, 1972.
Szasz, T. (ed.) *The Age of Madness*. New York: Doubleday, 1973.
Ullman, L.R., and Krasner, L. *Case Studies in Behavior Modification*. New York: Holt, Rinehart, & Winston, 1965.
Valenstein, E.S. *Brain Control: A Critical Examination of Brain Stimulation and Psychosurgery*. New York: Wiley, 1973.
Visher, J.S., Visotsky, H., and Waggner, R.W. APA's committee controversy—A rebuttal. *Psychiatric News*, November 21, 1973.

Vonnegut, K., Jr. *Player Piano.* New York: Holt, Rinehart, & Winston and Avon Library, 1967.
Vonnegut, K., Jr. *The Sirens of Titan.* New York: Dell, 1959.
Warren, J. Peace pills for presidents? *Psychology Today,* October 1973, pp. 59-60.
Weil, A. *The Natural Mind.* Boston: Houghton Mifflin, 1973.
Wright, A.T. *Islandia.* New York: Holt, Rinehart, & Winston, 1958.
Wyatt vs. Stickney (1971), 325, F. Supp. 781 (MD ALA 1971).
Wyatt vs. Stickney (1972), 344, F. Supp. 373 (MD ALA 1972).

Subject Index

Author Index